THE HEALTH HANDBOOK: A CONCISE GUIDE FOR COLLEGE STUDENTS

THE HEALTH HANDBOOK: A CONCISE GUIDE FOR COLLEGE STUDENTS

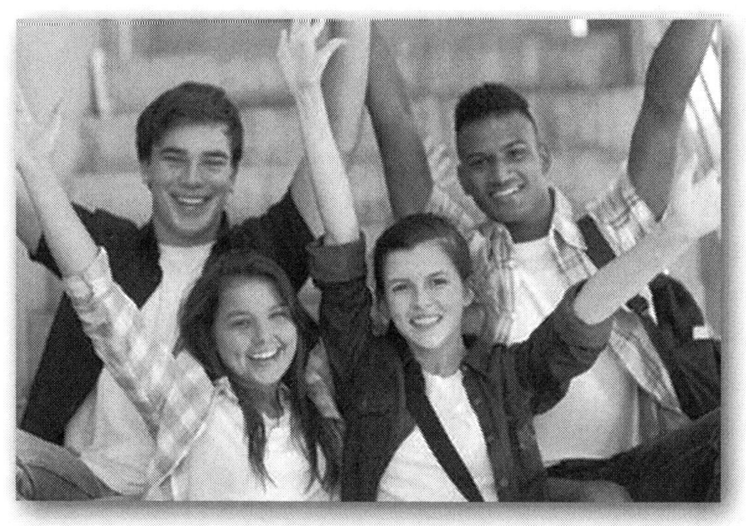

Dianna M. Jones
Doctor of Nursing Practice
Family Nurse Practitioner

ISBN: 1518806856
ISBN 13: 9781518806858
Library of Congress Control Number: 2015917878
CreateSpace Independent Publishing Platform
North Charleston, South Carolina

Foreword

The Health Handbook: A Concise Guide for College Students explores important aspects of personal health including physical, emotional, social and spiritual well-being. This concise guide encourages and assists students to make proper health choices and gives them the necessary tools and information to improve their overall well-being. The book presents factual information specific to the many issues faced by college students today. The topics discussed in the handbook range from alcohol, eating disorders, exercise, mental health, nutrition, preventative health, sexuality, sleep hygiene and substance abuse. This guide is intended to provide college students with the necessary resources and tools to achieve good health in all of these areas. Promoting health and wellness during the college years is essential. With the proper skills, students can establish and maintain healthy lifestyle habits that support a life full of health and wellness. Information is powerful and the decisions young adults make at this time will ultimately set the stage for future health and happiness. Working to establish and maintain healthy habits today will help pave the way to a future full of possibilities. The Health Handbook offers a short, concise easy-to-read guide for young adults to reference important topics and be given the proper tools and resources necessary to take care of themselves throughout the college years and beyond.

Disclaimer

This guide is not intended to replace professional medical care. If you have questions or are in need of medical attention consult with a healthcare provider immediately. Resources have been added to this guide to provide supplemental material and helpful information. Please note that the websites listed in the chapter conclusions might change over time and may or may not be available or useful to you.

Acknowledgments

I would like to thank the many students I have worked with over the years. They are the true inspiration for this book, and the reason I love what I do. I owe a debt of gratitude to Dr. Antoinette Hays for her leadership, guidance, and encouragement. A special thanks to my editor Christopher Gainty for his insight and expertise. I would also like to thank my friends and colleagues who provided support, advice, and comments. Above all, I want to thank my amazing husband, whose unending support and encouragement have proved invaluable.

Dedication

This book is dedicated to my wonderful children, Madeline and Dylan, who keep me young and grounded. I hope this book encourages and inspires you both to make wise decisions during your college years and beyond.

Table of Contents

Foreword · · · v
Disclaimer · · · vii
Acknowledgments · · · ix
Introduction · · · xv
Health · · · 1
Alcohol & Substance Abuse · · · 4
Sexual Health · · · 14
Nutrition · · · 25
Exercise · · · 34
Eating Disorders · · · 40
Mental Health · · · 45
Sleep · · · 49
Mind-Body Health · · · 52
Complementary and Alternative Therapies (CAM) · · · 55
Preventative Health · · · 59
Dear Dianna Q&A · · · 64
Conclusion · · · 83
About the Author · · · 85
Endnotes · · · 87
Photo Credits/Shutterstock.com · · · 103

Introduction

Students who leave home for college experience many different emotions from anxiety, fear, sadness and loneliness to joy, determination, and the anticipation of an exciting new challenge. College life may cause stress at times, but it is often one of the most exciting experiences in a young adult's life.

While learning about and exploring this new world, remember to take good care of all aspects of your life and health. The topics discussed in this handbook range from alcohol, eating disorders, exercise, mental health, nutrition, preventative health, sexuality, sleep hygiene and substance abuse. Inside, you will find the necessary tools to achieve good health in all of these areas. Balance is the key to optimal health, and a holistic approach will ensure a proper mix of physical, psychological, social, and spiritual well-being.

As you embark on this new journey, it is important to keep in mind that now you are in charge of your own life. The decisions you make at this time will ultimately set the stage for future health and happiness. Embrace this opportunity to be the very best you can by making healthy choices. Endless opportunities await you, and working to establish and maintain healthy habits today will help pave the way to a future full of possibilities.

Health

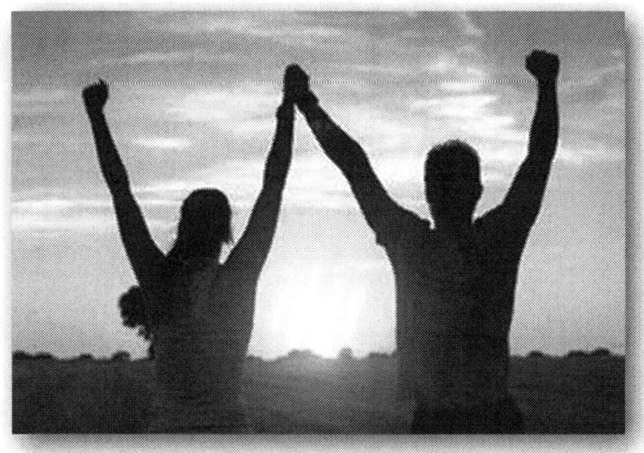

The World Health Organization defines "health" as "a state of complete physical, mental and social well-being and not merely the absence of disease or infirmity."[1] Health encompasses seven equally important categories: physical, mental/emotional, social, spiritual, intellectual, occupational and environmental.[2]

Physical health is a state of complete physical well-being enabling individuals to carry out their daily activities without discomfort or difficulty.[3] Examples include achieving fitness, maintaining adequate nutrition and proper body fat, avoiding risky sexual behaviors, refraining from drug, alcohol or tobacco use and in general, practicing positive lifestyle habits.

Mental/emotional health refers to a state of well-being in which individuals have the required cognitive and emotional abilities to function effectively in society on a day-to-day basis, managing the stresses which are a regular part of life, as well as feeling and expressing emotions such as happiness, sadness and anger in appropriate ways.[4]

Social health refers to the level of one's ability to interact successfully within a multicultural community, while showing respect for oneself and others. [5] Some examples include being able to effectively interact with people of other cultures, backgrounds and beliefs, cultivating and nurturing healthy relationships, as well as contributing and being present in the community.

Spiritual health describes the search for meaning in one's existence, a pursuit which can result in a life of purpose aligned to values and beliefs.[6] Ways to increase your spiritual well-being include exploring the many options for spiritual growth, being curious and asking questions and listening to your heart.[7]

Intellectual health refers to the cultivation of one's intellect and imagination and always striving to be the very best. Some examples include continuing with education, taking a course or learning something new that is challenging to you. It can also be as simple as reading a book for pleasure and being amongst others that challenge you intellectually.[8]

Occupational health includes one's ability to make use of their unique gifts and talents in the workplace. This includes finding a career that is meaningful and self-rewarding, while being able to balance work and personal time.[9]

Environmental health includes protecting the earth and its resources and adapting your surroundings to help you and others achieve a healthy lifestyle and quality of life. Examples include recycling, conserving water and minimizing your exposure to chemicals. [10]

Choosing to live a life of health and wellness in all the areas above gives balance and a sense of purpose and direction. Keep in mind that health and well-being are critical components not only to a successful college experience, but also for personal growth, healthy relationships, positive communication and social responsibility.[11]

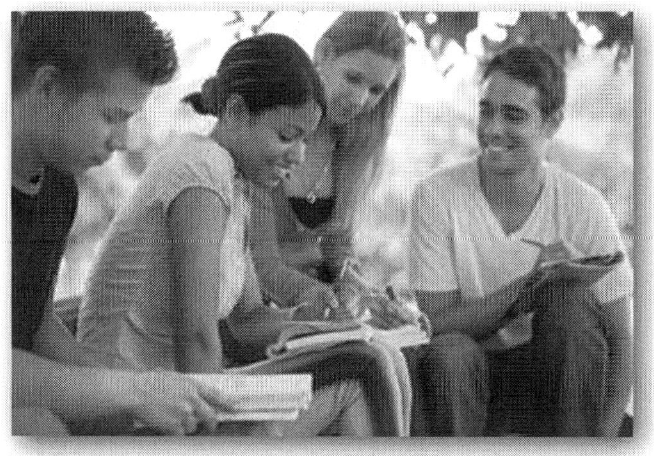

Alcohol & Substance Abuse

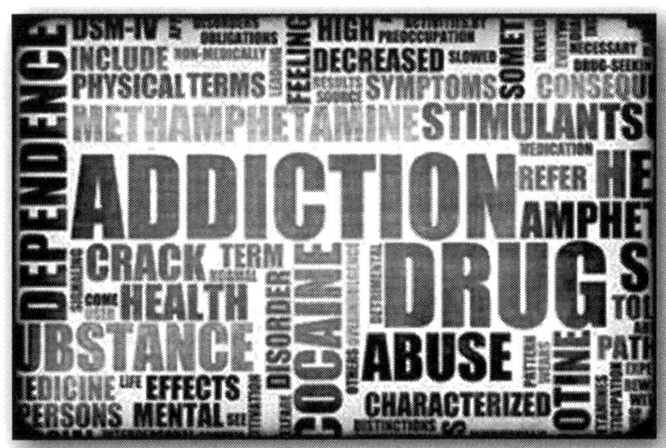

College is an exciting time and it presents an opportunity for growth, learning, socialization and self-discovery. Sadly, many college students waste much of their time experimenting with alcohol and drugs. This constitutes a significant problem on college campuses nationwide.[12]

Because young adults' brains continue to develop well into the college years, they face a greater risk of alcohol or drug dependency than the adult population.[13] Research shows that the most common drugs abused by college students today continue to be alcohol and tobacco, along with such substances as marijuana, cocaine, methamphetamines, GHB/Rohypnol (the "date rape" drug), ecstasy, heroin, bath salts and LSD.

ALCOHOL

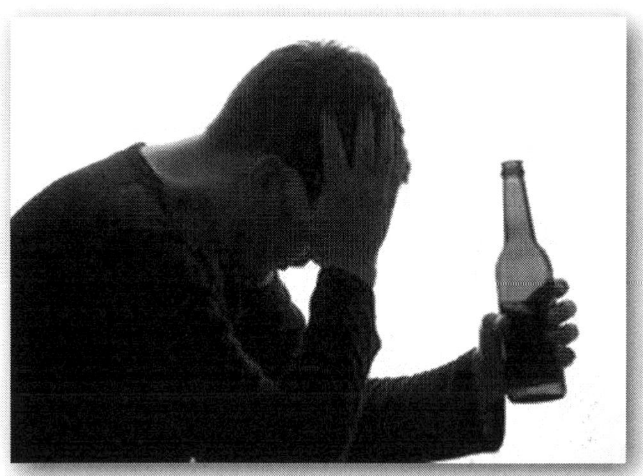

Alcohol is the most commonly abused substance on campuses, and it presents an ongoing health challenge for college students. Its consumption slows reaction time, dulls the senses and impairs judgment making it more difficult for the drinker to distinguish good decisions from bad ones. According to the National Institute on Alcohol Abuse and Alcoholism (NIAAA, 2013), approximately four out of five college students consume alcohol, and half of that number also report "binge" drinking, defined by the NIAAA as "drinking so much within about two hours that blood alcohol concentration (BAC) levels reach 0.08g/dL."[14]

Reference values for blood alcohol according to the Mayo Clinic:[15]

Not detected (Positive results are quantified)

Limit of detection: 10 mg/dL (0.01 g/dL)

Legal limit of intoxication is 80 mg/dL (0.08 g/dL)

Potentially lethal concentration: > or =400 mg/dL (0.4 g/dL)

Binge drinking can cause serious health issues and safety risks indeed; over the long term, excessive consumption of alcohol will lead to organ damage, especially, but not exclusively, to the liver.[16]

According to the National Institute of Health, some common consequences of alcohol abuse include: [17]

- **Academic Problems:** Every year, roughly 25% of college students report academic consequences of their drinking, including missed classes and a lower GPA.
- **Assault:** Every year, over 690,000 students between the ages of 18 and 24 are assaulted by another student who has been drinking.
- **Death:** 1,825 college students between the ages of 18 and 24 die each year from alcohol-related injuries such as motor vehicle crashes, drownings, falls, alcohol poisoning and other fatal accidents.[18]
- **Depression and Suicide Attempts:** Between 1.2 and 1.5 percent of students indicate that they have attempted suicide within the past year while under the influence of alcohol or other drugs.
- **Sexual Abuse:** More than 97,000 students between the ages of 18 and 24 are victims of alcohol-related sexual assault.

The notion that different forms of alcohol may have a greater or lesser effect on the body is false. Alcohol is the same, no matter what form it takes.[19] A 12 ounce can of beer, a 6 ounce glass of wine and a 1.5 ounce shot of hard liquor all contain roughly the same amount of alcohol. The difference is only in the concentration.[20]

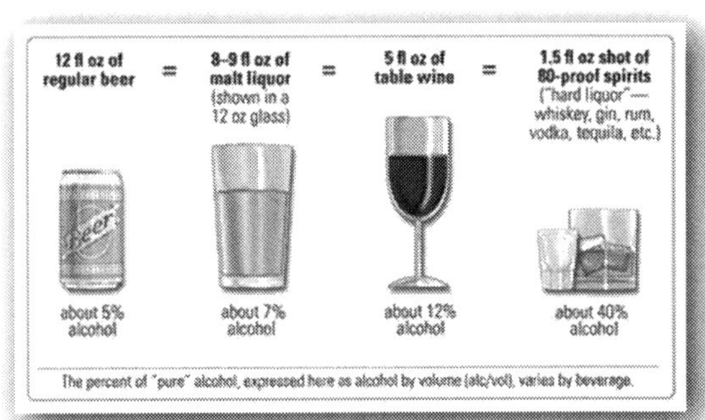

Courtesy of National Institute on Alcohol Abuse and Alcoholism (NIAAA, 2015)[21]

Remember, once consumed, alcohol takes time to metabolize and remains in your system for several hours. Drinking coffee, taking a cold shower, performing exercise or other activities will do nothing to sober you up, even if they make you feel more alert. You should also be aware that drinking on an empty stomach will allow the alcohol to enter your bloodstream much faster. It should also be noted that women absorb and metabolize alcohol differently than men.[22] Research has shown that women, in general, have lesser amounts of water in their bodies, and may also have a less active amount of the alcohol metabolizing enzyme ADH in their stomachs, "causing a larger proportion of the ingested alcohol to reach the blood" (NIAAA, 2013).[23] Therefore, women are more vulnerable to the adverse consequences of alcohol use, including liver and brain damage, heart disease, breast cancer and trauma.[24]

If your evening or weekend plans do happen to include drinking alcohol, be sure to have a trustworthy designated driver or some other means of transportation to bring you home safely. Also, never leave a friend behind that seems to have had too much to drink. In the event that medical attention is needed for alcohol intoxication, contact campus police or emergency medical services (EMS). Campus police or EMS would much rather receive your phone call and insure the safety of your friend than risk complications or death from alcohol poisoning or drug overdose.

DRUGS

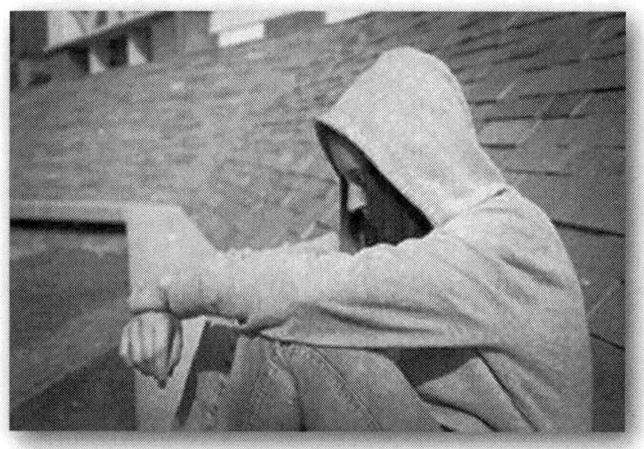

According to the National Survey on Drug Use and Health, in 2011, "the rate of current use of illicit drugs was 22.0 percent among full-time college students aged 18 to 22."[25] Illicit drug use not only poses long-term health problems such as addiction and changes in brain function, but it can also impact academic performance, learning, memory and judgment. If you or a friend are in need of services for issues resulting from the abuse of drugs, immediately seek help at your school's office of health services. There are numerous resources available today.

The list below presents the most common illicit drugs utilized on college campuses today:

Bath Salts - This drug is sold in small packets under such names as "Blue Wave," "Cloud Nine" and "White Lady."[26] Like LSD, it is a synthetic compound produced in a lab. Its use stimulates the central nervous system, and can lead to delusions, hallucinations, psychotic behavior and even death.[27]

Cocaine/Crack Cocaine - Both of these drugs are created from the coca plant but have a different level of refinement. Crack is a solid and it is heated and smoked, whereas cocaine is a powder and typically inhaled through the nose.[28] Cocaine stimulates the central nervous system and is felt almost immediately after having been ingested. Up to 75% of individuals who experiment with cocaine become addicted to the drug.[29] Users experience heart palpitations, dilated pupils, increased body temperature, and an increase in both heart rate and blood pressure. Continued use of cocaine may lead to chronic nasal congestion, chest pain, irregular heartbeat, cardiac arrest, breathing problems, headaches, abdominal issues, stroke, seizures, and in some cases, even death.

Hallucinogens - This category includes such drugs as LSD, PCP, psilocybin ("mushrooms") and others which interrupt a person's ability to understand and react quickly and appropriately to normal situations.[30] The user finds it difficult to think rationally and communicate effectively. These drugs often cause a person to perceive outside stimuli in a very unrealistic and disturbing way and as a result the user may often find him or herself in inappropriate and dangerous situations. This disconnection from reality can lead to bizarre, inappropriate, violent and sometimes even suicidal behaviors in the user.

Heroin - This drug is highly addictive and works by suppressing the central nervous system. Shortly after injecting, smoking or snorting heroin, the body experiences a feeling of euphoria, flushing of the skin, a dry mouth and a feeling of having "heavy" arms and legs.[31] Other short-term effects of heroin use include nausea and vomiting. Users of this drug suffer decreased mental function and risk a slowing of the user's respiratory rate to the point of failure.[32]

Marijuana - Marijuana consists of the leaves and buds of certain strains of the hemp plant. The user usually smokes it, either in a hand-rolled cigarette or from a pipe, but it may also be eaten or used to brew tea. Marijuana can cause respiratory problems, impaired memory and concentration, heart palpitations, depression, anxiety and panic attacks.[33] According to the National Institute on Drug Abuse, frequent marijuana use by young adults negatively impacts memory, learning and thinking. These effects can be long lasting and even permanent.[34]

MDMA (Ecstasy) - MDMA commonly referred to ecstasy or Molly is a synthetic drug which has both stimulant and psychedelic effects. It is usually taken in pill form, and first became widely known for its use at nightclubs. The effects of this drug last between four and six hours, and can include confusion, depression, anxiety, sleeplessness and paranoia. Users may also experience muscle tension, nausea, blurred vision, a feeling of faintness, tremors, rapid eye movement and sweating or chills. Ecstasy users risk dehydration, hyperthermia ("heat-stroke") and heart or kidney failure, and research has shown that the use of this drug also causes damage to parts of the brain critical to thought and memory.[35]

Methamphetamine - "Meth" or "Crystal Meth" is extremely addictive. It is usually injected, snorted or smoked and stimulates the central nervous system. Methamphetamine can be found in powdered form, similar to granulated crystals; in the form of a rock (known as "ice"); or, less commonly, in liquid form. Users initially experience an intense rush, along with such side effects as violent behavior, anxiety, confusion, sleep issues, hallucinations and mood swings.[36] Heavy use may also cause cardiovascular damage.

Rohypnol ("Roofies") – The "Date Rape" Drug - Rohypnol is one common brand name used to market flunitrazepam. Commonly known as "roofies", this drug slows the body's response to stimuli, causing sedation, amnesia and muscle relaxation. These reactions are felt within 20-30 minutes of taking the drug, and can last for a number of hours. The drug is often slipped into drinks surreptitiously, and leaves the person ingesting it slow to realize a threating situation as it develops. Too often, the person dosed becomes unable to remain alert enough to make wise choices in response. Such a situation can leave the person helpless in the face of unwanted sexual advances, increasing their risk of STIs, pregnancy, and physical and psychological trauma. In some cases, rohypnol can lead to decreased respiratory function, aspiration, and even death.[37] To assure safety, attend parties or other social gatherings with friends whom you trust. Remain aware of your surroundings, and watch out for one another. NEVER leave a friend alone if he or she appears to be under the influence of alcohol or drugs and never leave your drink unattended, even for a very short time. Also, avoid sharing someone else's drink and drinking from a punch bowl.

According to the National Council on Patient Information (NCPI), alcohol tops the list of substances abused on college campuses. However, the abuse of prescription drugs, such as stimulants, sedatives and pain relievers, represents a current and growing problem. Research shows that one in four students illegally use prescription medications.[38] In addition to possible addiction, the risk of using prescription stimulants such as Ritalin or Adderall can cause an elevation in blood pressure, heart rate and body temperature.[39] They also contribute to decrease sleep and appetite. Prolonged or repeated use can cause hostile behaviors and paranoia and at high doses, stimulants cause serious health issues including cardiovascular problems and stroke.[40] It is crucial that students neither share any of their own prescription drugs (especially medications for conditions such as depression, anxiety, insomnia or ADHD) nor use any medication prescribed to another person. Only a licensed medical professional has both the knowledge and prescription authority to determine who should be taking these drugs and the ability to make them available to that person by prescription.

TOBACCO

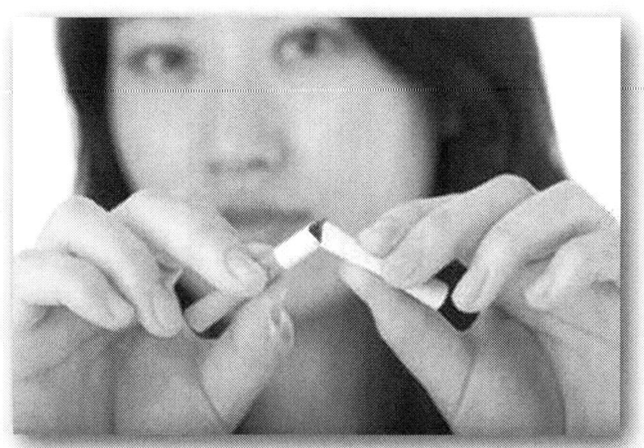

According to the American College Health Association (ACHA), students of colleges across the United States are taking steps to make their campuses smoke-free and as a result, many campuses are banning smoking, both indoors and outdoors.[41] Nevertheless, too many college students still smoke. According to the Department of Public Health, smoking continues to be the single most important factor increasing Americans' risk of heart disease, cancer and respiratory diseases.[42] If you do smoke, quitting is the right decision for many reasons. According to the Great American Smokeout (2012):[43]

1. Quitting reduces the risk of coronary artery disease later in life.
2. Quitting reduces the risk of lung cancer, emphysema, and other lung diseases.
3. Quitting will make it possible to climb stairs and walk without being out of breath.

4. Quitting will reduce or banish altogether the infamous "smoker's cough."
5. Quitting will allow you more energy to pursue the physical activities you enjoy most.
6. Quitting will make the money you save available for other needs.
7. Quitting will give you more control over your life.

When you are ready here are four tips which will help you to quit:

1. Get your mind ready and set a quit date.
2. Be sure to have plenty of support and encouragement from family, friends, classmates and support groups.
3. Learn new skills and develop new habits in order to distract yourself from the desire to smoke.
4. If you are given medication to help you quit, be sure to follow the directions for its use. Ask your healthcare provider about prescription and over-the-counter medications which are available and can aid in quitting smoking.

Be prepared for possible relapses or other challenges along the way. Most occur during the first three months of an attempt to quit and many people find it necessary to try several times before they are finally able to stop smoking for good. It is important not to allow these initial setbacks to deter you from quitting.

CONCLUSION

The abuse of drugs and/or alcohol has significant effects on the mind and body. Be sure to fully understand the facts about consuming drugs, tobacco or alcohol and how these substances can negatively impact your life and your college experience. If you are concerned about your alcohol and/or drug use, or are concerned about a friend, seek help from a medical professional immediately. Untreated, the complications arising from the abuse of drugs and alcohol can put the user and/or others at risk for serious harm.[44]

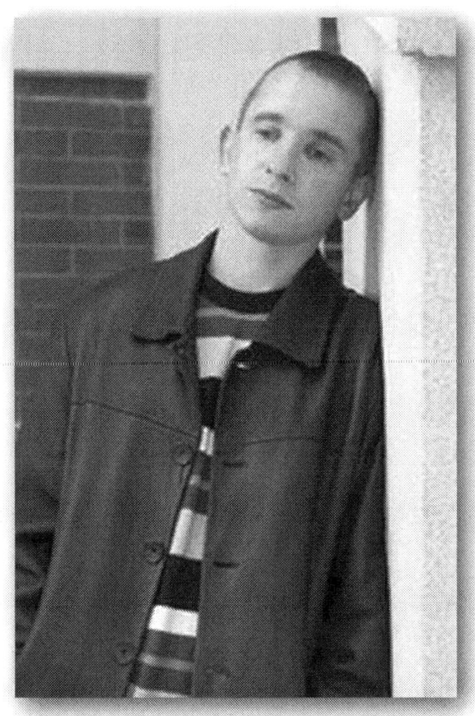

For additional information on the topics discussed in this chapter, see the Q&A section on page 64 and the resources below:

http://www.drugabuse.gov/

http://www.samhsa.gov/Treatment/

http://www.drugfree.org/

http://www.cdc.gov/TOBACCO/

http://www.cdc.gov/tobacco/data_statistics/fact_sheets/cessation/quitting/

http://smokefree.gov/

Sexual Health

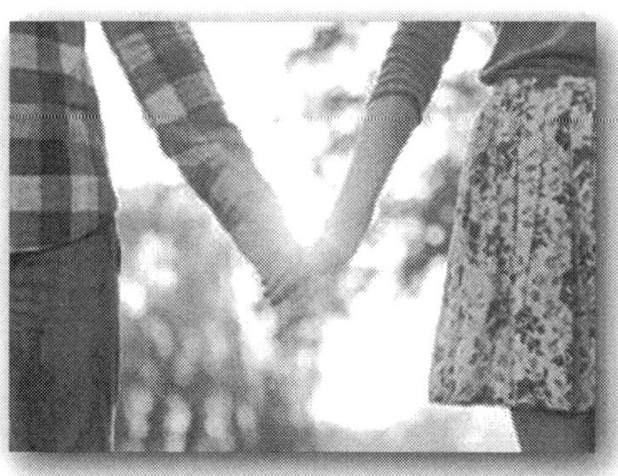

During the college years many students engage in sexual exploration.[45] Sexuality is a natural and healthy part of life, and open communication with your partner is vital to a successful relationship. It is crucially important that your partner respect you and honor your wishes, including your choice to refrain from sexual activity if that is your decision. Knowing and communicating your limits is an important prerequisite for a healthy, consensual relationship.

Ask yourself the questions below to help you determine if you are in a healthy relationship:

- Do you feel safe, secure and comfortable?
- Do you resolve your conflicts in a reasonable manner?
- Do you and your partner enjoy your time with one another?
- Do each of you take an interest in the other's life?
- Do you trust one another?
- Do you have sexual relations by choice?

Qualities such as respect, kindness and trust are important factors in maintaining a healthy relationship. Warning signs for an unhealthy relationship include controlling, mentally abusive, physically abusive or disrespectful behaviors and pressure to engage in sexual activity. You should end any relationship in which these behaviors appear.

Mutual respect is critically important to maintaining a healthy relationship. You and your partner should decide together whether or not sex is right for you.

"Sexual health" is much more than deciding whether or not to engage in sexual activity. Ask yourself about your own values and hopes for the future and try to determine how becoming sexually active might affect them. For example, there are many personal or religious reasons for which individuals decide to abstain from sexual activity. Some faith traditions forbid the use of contraception, or require waiting until marriage before becoming sexually active. If you are conflicted due to your religious or personal beliefs, you may find it helpful to discuss this issue with a trusted friend, counselor, healthcare provider or member of your clergy.

Students may also be conflicted or struggling with their sexual orientation. Research suggests that during the college years, students find it easier to explore and be open about their identity and interests.[46, 47] Most colleges have groups or resource centers for gay, lesbian, bisexual, transgender (GLBT) students.

Regardless of your sexual orientation, if you decide to become sexually active, there are several things to consider. Keeping yourself and your partner healthy and free of disease is vital. Researchers have identified approximately 25 different sexually transmitted diseases or infections (STDs or STIs). "The World Health Organization estimates that 250 million people in the world acquire an STD each year. In the United States, the number is 16 million."[48] And one in five college students have an STD.[49]

If you and your partner decide to become sexually active, you will need to protect yourselves from sexually transmitted diseases (STDs). STDs are caused by viruses, bacteria, protozoa and insects.[50] They are transmitted by sexual behaviors, and your risk of contracting an STD increases along with the number of partners with whom you engage in sexual activity. According to the Center for Disease Control (CDC), other than abstinence, the correct use of a male or female latex condom is the best way to protect yourself and your partner.[51] For proper use of these methods visit the CDC website: http://www.cdc.gov/condomeffectiveness/brief.html.

STDs continue to be a health challenge today, especially on college campuses. Research estimates that amongst the 16 million new cases of STDs occurring annually in the United States, 50% affect those between the ages of 15 and 24.[52]

STDs can cause both short term and long term problems that affect your overall well-being, including reproductive health problems such as infertility and ectopic pregnancy.[53]

SEXUALLY TRANSMITTED DISEASES (STDS)

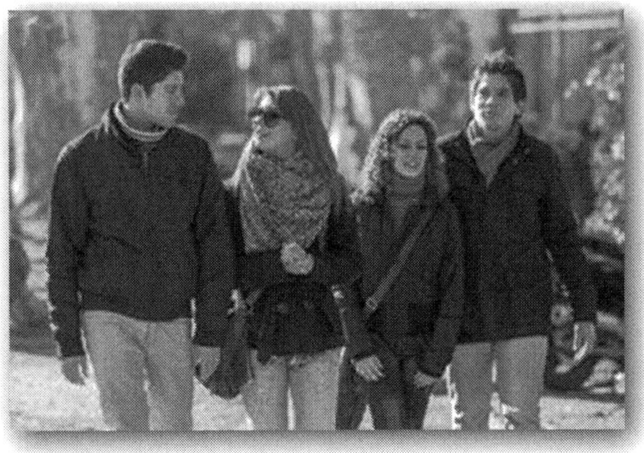

STD Quick Tips

- *Open communication*
- *Monogamy*
- *Always protect yourself*
- *Regular check-ups*
- *STD testing*

Information on the most common sexually-transmitted infections amongst college students today is listed below in order of prevalence of the disease:[54]

Human Papillomavirus (HPV)/Genital Warts – According to the CDC, Human Papillomavirus (HPV), the virus that causes cervical cancer and genital warts, is the most commonly experienced STD in the United States, affecting roughly 79 million Americans, with 14 million new cases every year. The CDC recommends HPV vaccination for all women younger than 26, and all men younger than 21. The HPV vaccine is most effective if individuals are immunized before engaging in sexual activity.[55] There are over 40 types of this virus that can infect the genital areas of both men and women and in some cases the mouth and throat. The vaccine protects against the most commonly experienced types of HPV, those which can leave the person afflicted and with an increased level of vulnerability for venereal diseases and cancer, including most cervical cancers.[56] Genital warts can present as a small bump, or as several bumps clustered together in the genital area. They may be large or small and are often described as looking like cauliflower. The warts appear anywhere from one week to several months after exposure to the virus from an infected partner. However, the varieties of HPV that cause genital warts are different from those that may lead to cervical cancer. The carcinogenic strains do not have the same symptoms and can only be detected through cervical screening. For this reason, it is vitally important for all women over the age of 21 who are sexually active or may have been exposed to an infected partner to be screened.[57] According to the CDC, "Most men who get HPV (of any type) never develop any symptoms or health problems." However, some research suggests that certain types of HPV may cause cancers of the penis, anus, or oropharynx (back of the throat, including base of the tongue and tonsils).[58]

Chlamydia – According to the CDC, chlamydia is one of the most common STDs, with approximately 1,441,789 cases reported in 2015. In women, the symptoms include abnormal vaginal discharge and a burning sensation during urination. Chlamydia can also cause sexual intercourse to be painful, and untreated infections can spread into the uterus and fallopian tubes, causing pelvic inflammatory disease.[59] Most men do not exhibit any symptoms of infection, although, some may experience a discharge from the penis, occasional pain and/or swelling in one or both testicles.

Gonorrhea – This STD can cause infections in the genital area, rectum and throat. Most men and women infected with gonorrhea will experience painful urination, discharge from the penis or vagina, and/or vaginal bleeding in women or painfully swollen testicles in men.[60]

Herpes – The herpes simplex virus responsible for this disease has two types: HSV-1, the virus that causes cold sores, and HSV-2, the virus more commonly found in the genital area. However, HSV1 can present in the genital area due to unprotected oral sex. Symptoms of infection include irritation, burning, itching, painful urination and tenderness in the genital area, along with multiple, painful open sores. Some may experience a fever and/or swollen lymph nodes. Recurrences of HSV are milder than the initial breakout, and present as scattered sores on the genital area. Research shows that approximately 1 in 5 college students in the United States have been exposed to HSV-2.[61]

Syphilis – This bacterial infection is on the rise in college age males.[62] It initially presents with a painless open sore known as a "chancre," which typically appears at day 21of exposure, but can range anywhere from day 10 to 90.[63] If the infection is not treated during that time frame, the sore heals, and the disease enters the second stage. This is characterized by such symptoms as skin rash, hair loss and circular, flat growths on the body. If the infection is left untreated, it can lay dormant and then reappear in a final stage called the tertiary stage, causing damage to major organs including the brain and heart.[64]

Trichomoniasis – This parasitic infection is considered the most common treatable STD.[65] The CDC estimates 3.7 million people in the United States have Trichomoniasis, although only about 30% ever develop symptoms. Some women may experience vaginal redness, irritation and swelling, along with a yellow-green discharge. Men may experience itching or irritation inside the penis, burning after urination or ejaculation, and/or discharge from the penis.[66]

Human Immunodeficiency Virus (HIV) – This virus attacks the body's immune system and destroys the cells (CD4) which fight infections and diseases, leaving the body unprotected. HIV was first identified over 30 years ago, and to date, millions around the world have died from the disease it causes, known as Acquired Immune Deficiency Syndrome (AIDS). Research continues, and while many advances have been made, no cure yet exists for AIDS. Researchers have developed new therapies that allow a greater number of people to live with the disease, sometimes holding it at bay for years. However, it remains a vicious killer. Exposure to HIV does not necessarily mean you will develop AIDS. Nevertheless, if you plan to be sexually active, it is vital that you know your status and that of your partner.

Pelvic Inflammatory Disease (PID) – Pelvic inflammatory disease is an infection of the female reproductive organs.[67] It is typically caused by complications from other STDs such as chlamydia and gonorrhea. PID may cause abdominal and pelvic pain, pain during sexual intercourse and vaginal discharge. Some women do not experience any symptoms at all, but may still be at risk for complications in a future pregnancy, as well as scar tissue, ectopic pregnancy and/or infertility.[68]

Hepatitis – Hepatitis refers to a group of viral infections that cause inflammation of the liver. The most common types are Hepatitis A, Hepatitis B and Hepatitis C. Hepatitis B is highly contagious and is typically contracted through sexual activity. It can also be passed through direct contact with blood, saliva, semen and vaginal secretions of an infected person. Research indicates that Hepatitis B is 50-100 times more infectious than HIV.[69] Vaccination is the best way to protect yourself against this STD.

Bacterial Vaginosis (BV) – BV is not considered an STD; however, it can be transmitted through sexual activity. BV is an overgrowth of one or more bacteria, causing an imbalance in the vagina and producing inflammation and vaginal discomfort. Other symptoms include a strong smelling, thin white vaginal discharge. Men do not get BV, but may serve as carriers of the bacteria responsible, and may infect their partners during sexual contact.

If you have had unprotected sex and are concerned about STDs, or are having any symptoms, be sure to visit your college's office of health services as soon as possible. Do not wait. Some untreated STDs can lead to serious health problems including pain and infection in other areas of the body and infertility.[70] Additionally, never treat yourself before being seen by a healthcare provider. Remember, when it comes to choosing whether or not to engage in sexual relations, you are in charge! If you are nervous or have questions, don't be shy. You deserve answers from your partner and/or a healthcare provider.

PREGNANCY

Research shows that due to the prevalence of unsafe sexual practices, women between the ages of 20 and 24 have the highest rate of unintended pregnancy. According to the CDC's latest research, approximately 80% of all college females are engaging in sexual activity.[71] CDC reports, 273,105 teen girls aged 15–19 years gave birth in 2013.[72] According to the National Campaign to Prevent Teen and Unplanned Pregnancy, "unplanned pregnancy and childbearing are also implicated in the failure of many young women to finish their college education. Research shows that 61% of women who have children after enrolling in community college fail to finish their degree, which is 65% higher than the rate for those who didn't have children."[73] Unintended pregnancy presents many obstacles for college students. Not only can it impact academic performance, postpone or disrupt educational goals, but it can also cause financial and emotional stress. The consequences of unintended pregnancy are significant, and the decision to become sexually active should be thought through carefully and completely.

Several methods to prevent unwanted pregnancy exist. The effectiveness of the methods available for protection vary (see chart) and are listed in order of efficacy.[74]

Statistics courtesy of the Center for Disease Control and Prevention (CDC) on typical efficacy rates with respect to pregnancy (percentages indicate per 100 users per year):[75]

Methods (listed most effective to least)	**Typical Use Efficacy Rates**
Abstinence	100%
Male Sterilization (Vasectomy)	99.85%
IUD (Intrauterine Device) Hormonal	99.8%
Implant	99.5%
Female Sterilization (Abdominal, Laparoscopic, Hysteroscopic)	99.5%
IUD (Intrauterine Device) Copper	99.2%
Injection	94%
Oral Contraceptives	91%
Diaphragm or Cervical Cap	88%
Male Latex Condom	82%
Female Condom	79%
Withdrawal Method	78%
Natural Family Planning or Fertility Awareness	76%
Sponge	76% (women without children) 88% (women with children)
Spermicides	72%

For more detailed information on any of the methods listed, visit the CDC website at http://www.cdc.gov/reproductivehealth.

Unplanned pregnancy can cause significant obstacles for college students and there is certainly a lot to consider when becoming sexually active. Before you engage in any sexual behavior, speak with a trusted healthcare provider. He or she will be able to explain the many options of protection that are currently available, and help you to decide which is best suited for you.

SEXUAL ASSAULT

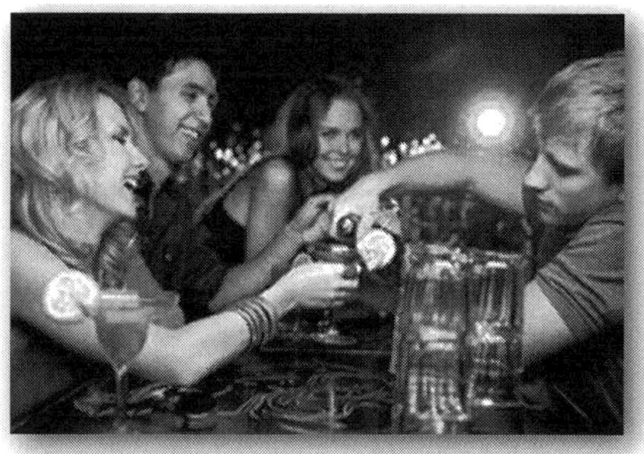

Sexual Assault Quick Tips

- *Trust your instincts*
- *Form a buddy system*
- *Responsible drinking*
- *Avoid being alone*
- *Never leave your friends*

Sexual assault is defined as an assault of a sexual nature on another person without their consent. Sexual assault is against the law and it includes a wide range of unwanted sexual contact such as:

- forced vaginal, anal or oral penetration
- forced sexual intercourse
- inappropriate touching
- forced kissing
- child molestation
- exhibitionism and/or voyeurism
- obscene phone calls
- torture of a victim in a sexual manner

Research shows that the majority of reported assaults in the average college population involve drugs and alcohol. "As many as one in four women experience unwanted sexual intercourse while attending college in the United States" with many of these events happening at or after parties.[76] According to the CDC, in a national survey of adults, "nearly 1 in 5 (18.3%) women and 1 in 71 men (1.4%) reported experiencing rape at some time in their lives." Of this group, "37.4% of female rape victims were first raped between ages 18-24. In a study of undergraduate women, 19% experienced attempted or completed sexual assault since entering college."[77]

There are several things you can do to protect yourself and avoid sexual assault. At parties, use caution when choosing to consume punches or other pre-mixed drinks, as you can neither be sure of the alcohol content of the drink nor whether other substances may have been added. Never leave your drink unattended, and watch out for a friend who seems to have had too much to drink. If you and a group of friends are out, it is safer to remain together as a group, and watch out for each other. Know when it is time to leave, and trust your gut instincts about anyone or any situation that does not seem right to you.

Most who have experienced sexual assault blame themselves, but it is never the victim's fault. If you or someone you know has been a victim of a sexual assault on campus, immediately seek treatment from your college's office of health services or the nearest hospital emergency room. You should give a full report of the incident to campus police, or if you are off campus, to the local police department. Do not touch or change any part of the scene where the assault took place, and unless medically necessary, you should not wash or wipe clean any part of your body or remove or change your clothing.[78] This will allow hospital staff to effectively collect evidence on your behalf.

CONCLUSION

Becoming sexually active comes with considerable responsibilities. You owe it to yourself to fully understand how sex will affect your social and academic life and your health. If you are sexually active or plan to become sexually active, consult with a healthcare provider to discuss your options for protection against STDs and unwanted pregnancy.

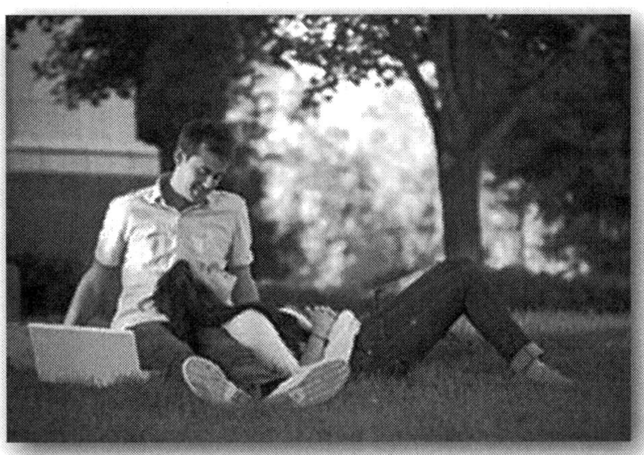

For additional information on the topics discussed in this chapter, see the Q&A section on page 64 and the resources below:

http://www.cdc.gov/features/collegehealth/
http://www.youngwomenshealth.org/
http://www.bacchusnetwork.org/sexual-health.html
http://www.nsvrc.org/
http://www.cdc.gov/ViolencePrevention/pdf/SV-DataSheet-a.pdf
http://www.apa.org/helpcenter/sexual-orientation.aspx
http://www.cdc.gov/lgbthealth/youth-programs.htm
http://www.glbtnationalhelpcenter.org/hotline/index.html

Nutrition

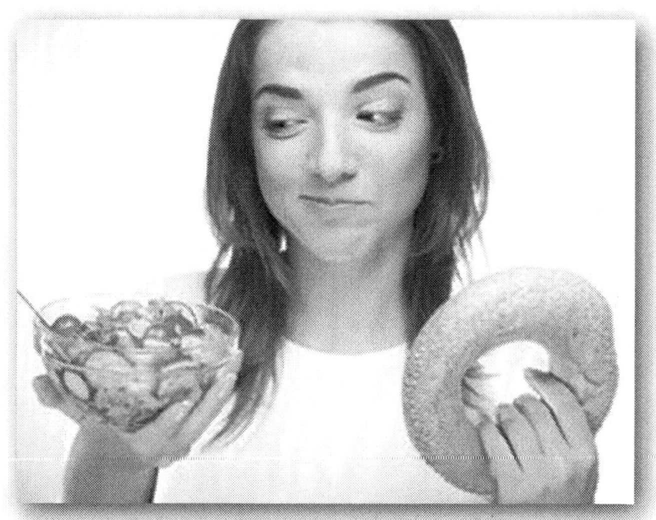

Eating on a college campus may seem challenging because of the many choices, but healthy eating does not have to be compromised or complicated if you keep familiar nutrition standards in mind. According to a study conducted by Zagorsky and Smith (2011), women gain an average of 2.4 pounds during their freshman year and men an average of 3.4 pounds.[79] Unhealthy habits that contribute to weight gain include consuming high-calorie vending machine food and soda, skipping meals and/or binge eating, and drinking too many alcoholic beverages. Lack of aerobic exercise also contributes to weight gain.

You may remember the classic "food pyramid" intended to indicate the types and amounts of each food group found in an optimal diet. More recently, this symbol has been replaced by a colorful plate of food. The plate displays four sections, with one half made up of fruits, vegetable and healthy oils and the other half representing proteins, grains and dairy.

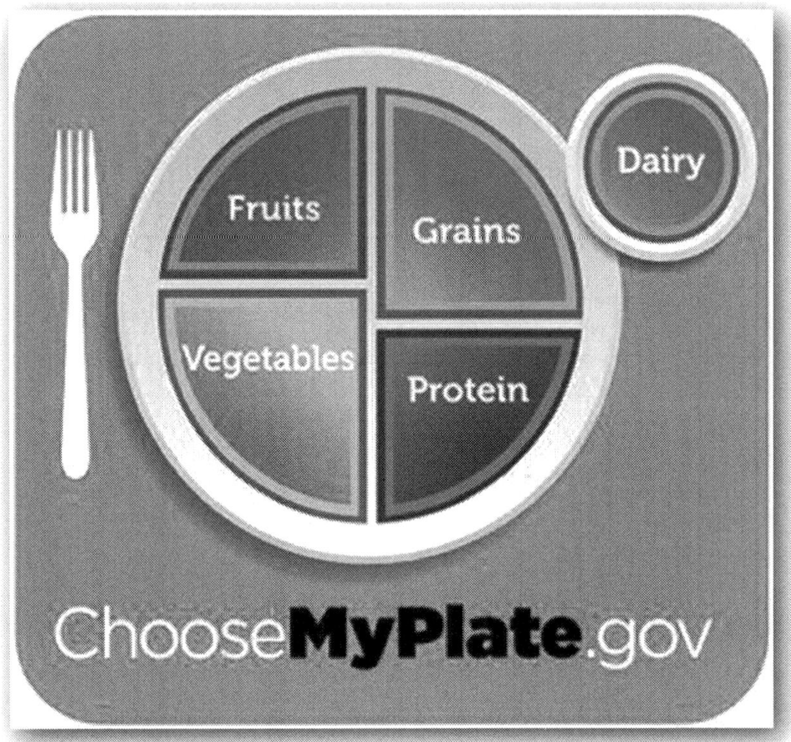

Courtesy of United States Department of Agriculture[80]

There is no need to measure out serving sizes, as long as this chart is used as a guide when making choices at each meal.[81] Vegetables and fruits should take up half of your plate (with the veggie portion being a bit bigger), and grains and protein foods should take up the other half (with more grains on this side). Foods such as fruits, vegetables and whole grains are central to healthy eating. These are "good carbohydrates" and they help to keep your blood pressure and blood sugar stable, which in turn helps keep your weight under control. On the other hand, "bad carbohydrates" such as sugar and foods prepared using white flour (such as white breads and cakes) can increase your risk of diabetes, heart disease and weight gain.

Calcium is another important nutrient needed for strong bones and essential to the proper function of your heart, muscles and nerves. When calcium levels are low, our bodies are programmed to automatically take calcium from our bones, causing them to weaken.[82] Calcium is found in milk and milk products, fish, meats, beans, nuts, fruits, vegetables, bread and cereals. Vitamin D is needed to absorb calcium in the body and good sources of vitamin D include traditional, almond or soy milk, fortified breakfast cereals, high-fat fish such as salmon and mackerel, egg yolks, oysters, and even daily exposure to 30 – 60 minutes of sunlight. The recommended daily allowance of calcium for adults of both genders is 1,000 mg.[83]

While eating healthy foods rich in vitamins and limiting unhealthy fatty foods is important, it is vital to remember that we also need a certain amount of fat in our diet every day. For example, of a 2,000 calorie-a-day diet, 400 to 700 calories can come from dietary fat, (between 44 and 78 grams of fat per day).[84] As there are 5 different types of fats, it is important to know which fats you are putting in your body in order to achieve a healthier diet. Below is a brief description of each type of fat:[85]

Monounsaturated fat – This is a good fat. It helps to reduce the amount of "bad" cholesterol in the blood (LDL) without decreasing the good cholesterol (HDL) levels. Foods high in this fat include peanuts, canola and olive oils, avocados and most nuts.

Polyunsaturated fat – This fat decreases the levels of both LDL and HDL found in the blood. Foods high in this fat include seeds and vegetable oils such as corn, safflower and soy.

Omega-3 fatty acids – These have been shown to help decrease the risk of coronary artery disease. Good sources include such foods as walnuts, salmon, herring and tuna.

Saturated fat – Saturated fat is usually solid at room temperature. Saturated fats are most commonly found in such dairy products as butter and ice cream, as well as in cocoa butter. These fats are known to clog arteries and contribute to coronary artery disease. Saturated fats are often found in many of our favorite foods, such as steak, butter, cheese and ice cream. Difficult though it may be, you should try to limit your intake of this fat.

Trans fat – Also known as "partially hydrated oil," these man-made fats can clog arteries if eaten in excess. This type of fat is most commonly encountered in such foods as french fries, onion rings and donuts.[86]

Students that maintain a vegetarian diet will need to be mindful when planning their meals and be sure to include certain nutrients the body needs to be healthy. Listed below are important nutrients and food sources recommended by the Mayo Clinic:[87]

- **Calcium** is essential for healthy teeth and bones. Food sources for calcium include milk, dairy, dark green vegetables such as broccoli and kale. Calcium enriched products including juices, yogurt, tofu and cereals are other good options.
- **Iodine** helps in the production of thyroid hormones regulating metabolism, growth and function of vital organs. Food sources for iodine include dried seaweed, cod, shrimp, baked potato, tuna in oil and boiled egg.[88]
- **Iron** is an important part of the blood cells. Sources of iron are found in beans, peas, lentils, dark leafy vegetables, dried fruits and enriched cereals.
- **Omega-3-fatty acids** are important for maintaining a healthy heart. Food sources include canola and soy oils, soybeans, ground flax seed and walnuts.
- **Protein** is vital for healthy skin, bones, muscles and organs. Sources of protein include dairy, eggs, soy products, nuts and legumes.
- **Vitamin B-12** is essential for red cell production and anemia prevention. Sources of B-12 are mostly found in animal products so it is recommended that vegetarians take a supplement. Some food sources for B12 include fortified products, eggs, Swiss cheese and low-fat dairy.[89]

- **Vitamin D** assists in bone health. In addition to sun light exposure, food sources of vitamin D include cow's milk, soy and rice milk and some cereals.
- **Zinc** assists with cell division and formation of proteins. [90] Food sources include cheese, dairy and soy products, nuts, wheat germ and legumes.

According to the Mayo Clinic there are several different types of vegetarian diets:[91]

- **Lacto-vegetarian diet** excludes meat, fish, poultry and eggs. Lacto-vegetarian includes dairy products such as cheese, yogurt, butter and milk into their diet.
- **Lacto-ovo vegetarian diet** excludes meat, fish and poultry, but includes eggs and dairy products.
- **Ovo-vegetarian diet** excludes meat, poultry, seafood and dairy products, but includes eggs into their diet.
- **Vegan diet** excludes meat, poultry, fish, eggs and dairy products and foods that contain animal products.

Regardless of your motivation for choosing to eat a vegetarian diet, you will need to be sure to eat enough of the recommended nutrients listed above. The importance of any healthy diet is understanding what you are consuming while enjoying the various food options available.

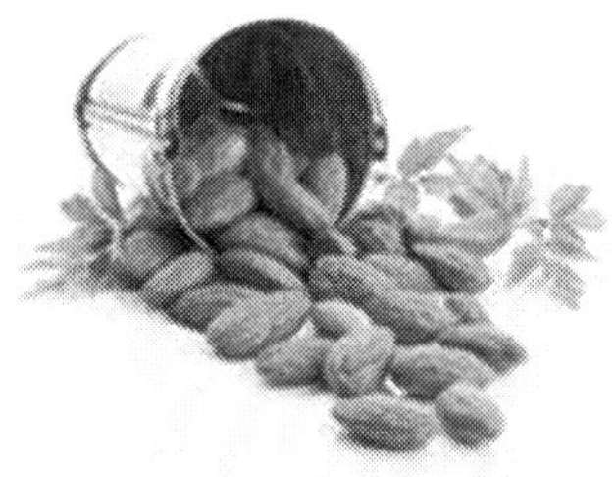

Listed below are some healthy food choices which should be available in your school's cafeteria or dining hall:

1. **Sweet potatoes** are loaded with carotenoids, vitamin C, potassium, and fiber.
2. **Grape tomatoes** are sweeter and firmer than regular tomatoes, and due to their smaller size, are perfect for snacking or dipping. They are packed with vitamin C, vitamin A, fiber and phytochemicals, all of which are important for staying healthy.
3. **Fat free cow's milk, almond or soy milk** are excellent sources of calcium, proteins and vitamins and have no artery-clogging fat or cholesterol.
4. **Eggs** contain an amazing amount of nutrients. Studies show that eating eggs for breakfast helps keep your hunger satisfied longer than consuming carbohydrates, such as pancakes, toast or donuts. One egg has all 9 essential amino acids, and contains 6 grams of protein.
5. **Blueberries** are rich in fiber, vitamin C and antioxidants.
6. **Nuts and seeds** are high in phytosterols, a substance which has been shown to lower cholesterol levels. Recommended nuts and seeds include sunflower seeds, pistachios, pumpkin seeds, pine nuts, and especially peanuts. Although high in fat and calories, research shows that a small serving of peanuts can be a great source of protein, as well as antioxidant polyphenols. And the healthy monounsaturated fats in peanuts are more easily metabolized by the body than are the saturated fats found in processed foods.
7. **Beans** are high in protein. Fava beans are full of flavonoids, a group of phytonutrients that have antioxidant and anti-inflammatory properties.[92] Packed with fiber and antioxidants, beans are not only low in "bad" cholesterol and calories but are also known for helping to minimize or prevent the occurrence of disease.
8. **Wild salmon** is rich in Omega-3 fatty acids, which studies have shown can help reduce the risk of heart attack and coronary artery disease by encouraging the body to burn fat. Wild salmon has 32%

fewer calories than farm-raised salmon and has healthy amounts of "good fats." A four ounce serving of wild salmon provides a full day's requirement of vitamin D, as well as vitamin B12, niacin and selenium, and is an excellent source of vitamin B6 and magnesium.[93]

9. **Crackers** are a good alternative to potato chips. Whole grain rye crackers are loaded with fiber, and are usually fat-free.
10. **Brown rice** is rich in fiber, magnesium, vitamin E, vitamin B-6, copper, zinc and phytochemicals. It also contains selenium, a trace mineral shown to significantly decrease the risk of colon cancer.[94]
11. **Apples** are low in calories, full of fiber, and can help to clean teeth, strengthen gums, decrease cholesterol levels and detoxify the body. Apples also have antiviral properties which help to keep you healthy and disease-free. They can also aid in digestion.[95]
12. **Oranges** are rich in vitamin C, vitamin A, calcium, potassium, and pectin.[96] Research shows that a diet high in citrus fruits provides statistically significant protection against both cardiac disease and some types of cancer.[97]
13. **Butternut squash** is a good source of vitamins and minerals. Each ½ cup serving has 5 grams of fiber and a substantial amount potassium, vitamin B6, vitamin A and vitamin C.
14. **Green vegetables** such as kale, spinach, green beans and broccoli are loaded with vitamin C, carotenoids, calcium, folate, potassium and fiber.

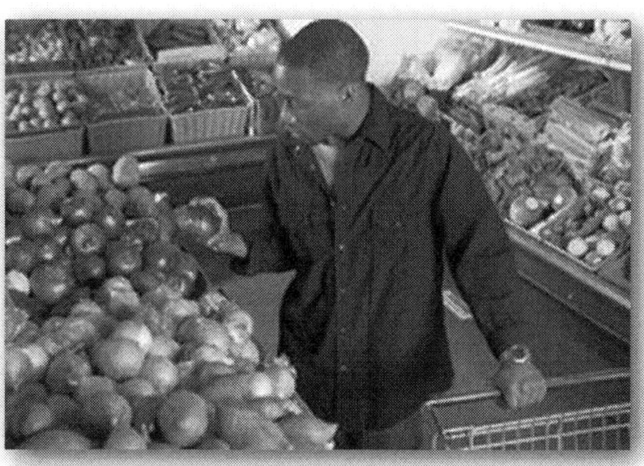

CONCLUSION

Whether in the cafeteria, the dining hall, at home or in a restaurant, vegetables should be an important part of your diet. As much as possible, eat grilled or baked foods, rather than foods which have been fried. When choosing carbohydrates, eat whole grains (e.g. whole grain bread, brown rice) as much as possible, and minimize your consumption of the refined flour found in white bread and white pasta. Drink low-fat or skim milk instead of whole milk or cream-based drinks. Drink lots of water, seltzer or fresh fruit juice instead of soda, energy drinks or other sweet drinks. Eat fruit or yogurt, and limit sweet desserts such as cakes, cookies or ice cream. Also, be aware of foods labeled "low fat" as they often have extra sugar.

The American Heart Association recommends that women consume no more than 100 calories per day of sugar (about six teaspoons or 25 grams), and that men consume no more than 150 calories per day, (nine teaspoons or 37.5 grams).[98] Eat plenty of fish and lean meats, and try to avoid portions which are higher in fat. Ideally you should eat between five and nine servings per day of fresh fruits and vegetables.

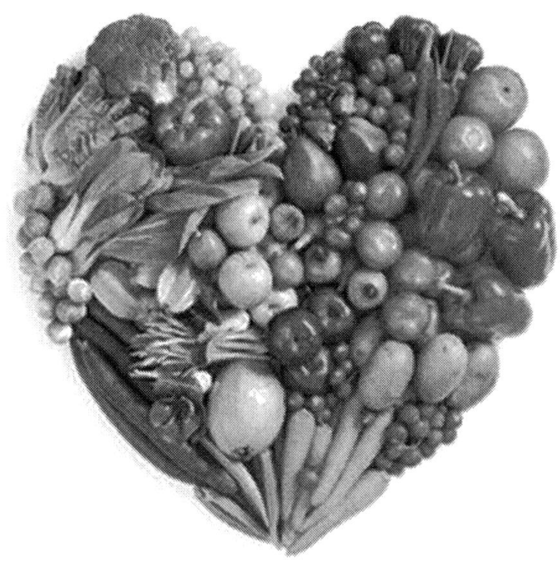

For additional information on the topics discussed in this chapter, see the Q&A section on page 64 and the resources below:

http://www.cdc.gov/healthyweight/healthy_eating/

http://www.choosemyplate.gov/healthy-eating-on-budget.html

http://www.nhlbi.nih.gov/health/public/heart/obesity/wecan/toolsresources/nutrition.htm

http://www.hsph.harvard.edu/nutritionsource/

http://www.webmd.com/diet/ss/slideshow-vegetarian-diet

http://www.fruitsandveggiesmorematters.org/cdc-resources

http://www.vrg.org/

Exercise

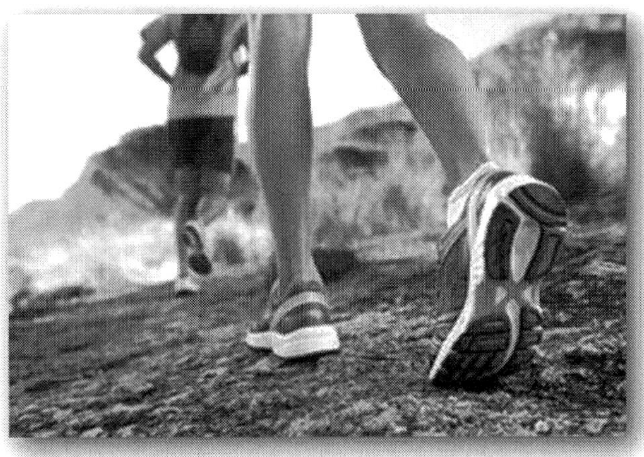

Physical activity is vital to staying healthy, especially any type of aerobic exercise such as walking, running, swimming or cycling.[99] Exercising at least three times per week is recommended for cardiac health, and will also help to control your weight, increase your energy level and contribute to your psychological well-being.

When choosing an exercise program, you need to keep in mind both your physical capabilities and your academic schedule. It is important that you choose a fitness activity that you enjoy, so that you will be motivated to reserve time in your schedule for exercise. For best results, you should vary your routine, both to provide your body with a more comprehensive workout and to avoid getting bored. Whatever exercise you choose, it is important that you know your body's limits.

The three main types of exercise are described below:

Aerobic exercise – Research has shown that this type of exercise is most beneficial for the body. Aerobic means "with oxygen," and refers to sustained physical exertion. This increases blood flow through the heart, the lungs and the large muscles. During aerobic exercise, you will breathe faster and deeper in order to provide your heart and other muscles with the oxygen they need in order to work harder.[100] Common aerobic exercises include jogging, power walking, cycling, swimming, skating or rowing.

Anaerobic exercise – Exercise intended primarily to increase muscle strength, rather than endurance, is referred to as "anaerobic," meaning "without oxygen." Anaerobic exercise consists of short, brief, strength-based exercises such as weight lifting. Due to the brief, intense nature of these activities, the muscles are unable to get enough oxygen to sustain the activity for prolonged periods of time. During anaerobic exercise, lactic acid builds up in the muscles, affecting their performance and causing fatigue and discomfort. For this reason, anaerobic exercise can only be done in short bursts.

Stretching exercise – This type of exercise is designed to improve flexibility and prevent injury. Stretching helps to preserve and in some cases increase a muscle group's range of possible motion, as well as strengthening and toning muscles, and improving stability and dexterity. When stretching, it is important to pay attention to the muscles in both one's upper and lower extremities.

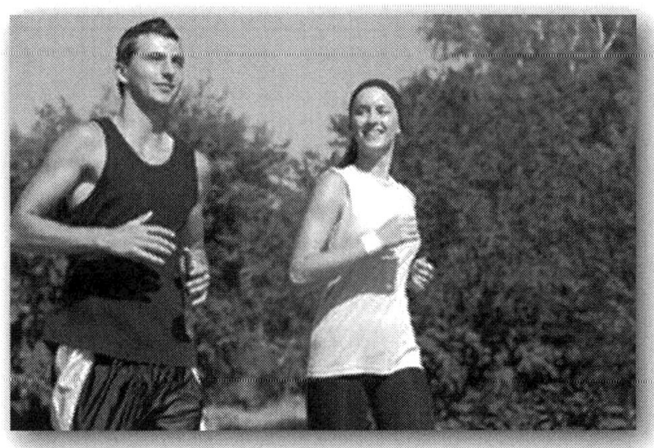

GETTING STARTED

As you begin to incorporate regular exercise into your daily routine, it is best to take it slowly, increasing the intensity, duration and frequency of your chosen activity gradually. Experts say that ideally, you should exercise at least three days per week for 30 minutes per session, but you may need to begin with a shorter workout, about 10-15 minutes.[101] As your body adjusts to the activity, you should gradually be able to work your way up to a 30-45 minute sessions. It is important that you give your body time to adjust so as to maximize the benefits to your health while not over doing it. For best results, it is recommended that your workout incorporate all three types of exercise listed.

No matter the routine you choose, you should always remember to warm up before exercising, and cool down when you are finished. Your warm-up should last at least five minutes, and should include stretching in order to both prepare your muscles for more vigorous activity and stimulate blood circulation.

Once you have finished your workout, it is also important that you cool down, slowing the heart from an active pace to its more usual rate. Exercise dilates blood vessels in order to allow for the increased blood flow and to supply the body with sufficient oxygen. Stopping abruptly can cause this larger-than-normal amount of blood to pool in the dilated blood vessels, changing the way the heart pumps and possibly leading to the unpleasant feeling of dizziness.[102] After finishing your workout, it is important to allow for five to ten minutes of reduced activity in order to return your heart rate to a calm state of 100-120 beats per minute.[103] To do this, it is a good idea to walk or do some mild stretching.

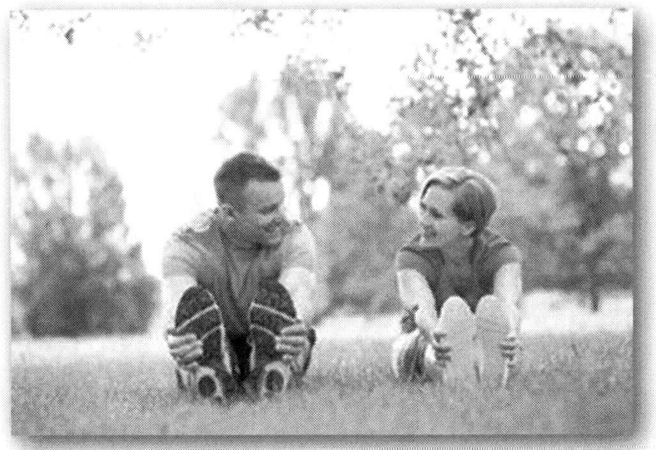

Below are listed some of the benefits of regular exercise:[104]

- **Increases your energy and endurance** - People who exercise on a regular basis gain additional energy, strength and endurance.
- **Strengthens and boosts your immune system** - Research shows that exercise improves the function of your immune system, enabling your body to fight off infection of environmental pathogens.
- **Reduces stress, depression and anxiety** - Research shows that exercise can reduce your level of stress and calm your worries, at least to some extent, helping you to relax.
- **Promotes better sleep** - Working out three to four times per week for at least 20 – 30 minutes will help you to both fall asleep more easily and sleep more soundly.

- **Improves confidence** – Knowing that you are actively working to improve your health through exercise is a wonderful way to increase your self-esteem and confidence.

In order for your fitness regimen to have the best results, it is important that you maintain a healthy diet and drink plenty of water. Staying hydrated is especially important. While exercising, watch for such symptoms of dehydration as headache, difficulty in concentrating, fatigue and dizziness. Dehydration can also increase your risk of kidney infections and cause constipation.

The FDA recommends that you drink at least eight glasses (two liters) of water per day, although some of that amount can come from equivalent amounts of coffee, tea, milk or fruit juices (alcoholic drinks cannot be counted).[105, 106] Water and drinks that contain water deliver oxygen and nutrients to different parts of the body, regulate body temperature through perspiration, reduce joint friction, facilitate movement, remove toxins and waste from the body, and act as a natural cushion for internal organs.[107]

CONCLUSION

In addition to offering interscholastic and intramural team sports, most college campuses also have fitness centers with exercise equipment such as weight machines, free weights, treadmills, stationary bikes, ellipticals, rowing machines and a track. Your college may also have a pool, and may offer a variety of physical fitness classes, such as weight training, martial arts, aerobics, yoga, and others. You should explore the options available, and decide which makes sense for you.

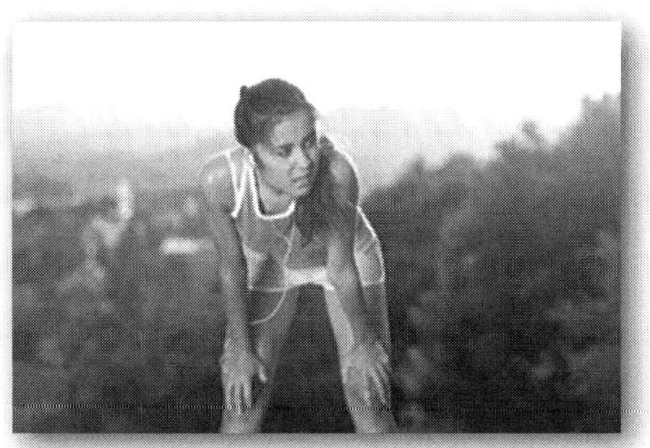

For additional information on the topics discussed in this chapter, see the Q&A section on page 64 and the resources below:

http://www.cdc.gov/physicalactivity/

http://www.nlm.nih.gov/medlineplus/exerciseandphysicalfitness.html

http://www.4collegewomen.org/fact-sheets/exercise.html

Eating Disorders

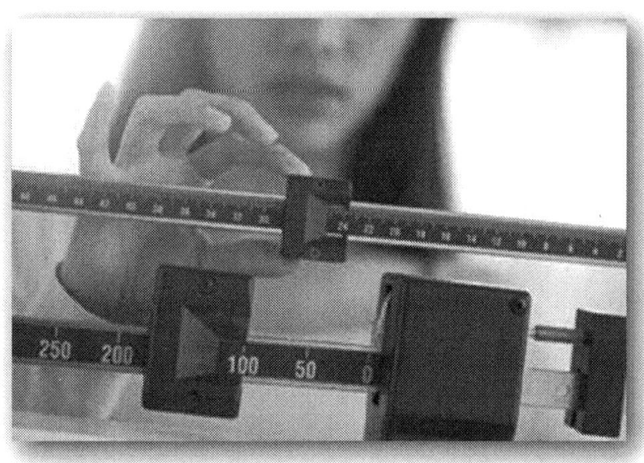

Eating disorders affect people of all ages. However, the research shows that they are especially common among teens and young adults.[108] There are many factors that can contribute to the development of an eating disorder including genetics, psychological or mental health problems, trauma, and societal and/or cultural norms.[109] The two main eating disorders that affect young adults are anorexia nervosa and bulimia nervosa.

Anorexia nervosa is an eating disorder characterized by weight loss to an extent considered unhealthy for the person's age and body type. Most people with anorexia obsess about their bodies, and have an unrealistic fear of gaining weight. They are unable to recognize what a healthy weight looks and feels like, and always feel a compulsive need to be thinner. Because of their fear, they will often starve themselves or make use of other unhealthy methods to lose weight. Anorexia nervosa is one of the most common psychiatric diagnoses in young women, and has the highest death rate of any mental health condition.[110]

By contrast, those suffering from **bulimia nervosa** will typically "binge eat" consuming excessive amounts of food and then attempt to eliminate the calories through either self-induced vomiting or the abuse of laxatives.

Common warning signs of anorexia nervosa and bulimia nervosa are listed below:[111]

Anorexia nervosa	**Bulimia nervosa**
• Dramatic weight loss. • Preoccupation with weight, food, calories, fat, and dieting. • Refusal to eat certain foods or categories of food (e.g. a refusal to eat carbohydrates). • Frequent complaints of feeling overweight, despite weight loss. • Anxiety about gaining weight. • Denial of hunger. • Development of food rituals (e.g. eating foods in certain orders, excessive chewing, rearranging food on a plate). • Excuses for avoiding mealtimes or situations involving food. • Excessive, rigid exercise regimen despite weather, fatigue, illness, or injury and the need to burn off calories taken in. • Withdrawal from usual friends and activities. • In general, behaviors and attitudes indicating that weight loss, dieting, and control of food are becoming primary, even obsessive concerns.	• Evidence of binge eating, including the discovery or finding empty wrappers and/or containers. • Evidence of purging behaviors, including frequent trips to the bathroom after meals; signs and/or odors of vomiting, presence of wrappers or packages of laxatives or diuretics. • Excessive, rigid exercise regimen despite weather, fatigue, illness, or injury and the compulsive need to burn off calories taken in. • Unusual swelling of the cheeks or jaw area. • Calluses on the back of the hands and knuckles from self-induced vomiting. • Discoloration or staining of the teeth. • Creation of lifestyle schedules or rituals to make time for binge-and-purge sessions. • Withdrawal from usual friends and activities. • In general, behaviors and attitudes indicating that weight loss, dieting, and control of food are becoming primary concerns.

Both conditions are very serious, and can be difficult to manage on one's own. Eating disorders can interfere with a person's social relationships and academic performance, in addition to physical well-being. Someone suffering from anorexia or bulimia may experience sadness, depression, anxiety, fear, guilt and hopelessness, along with such physical symptoms as fatigue, weakness, heart palpitations, menstrual issues and constipation.[112] If you believe that you, a roommate or a friend could possibly be suffering from an eating disorder, you should seek help from a healthcare provider immediately.

OBESITY

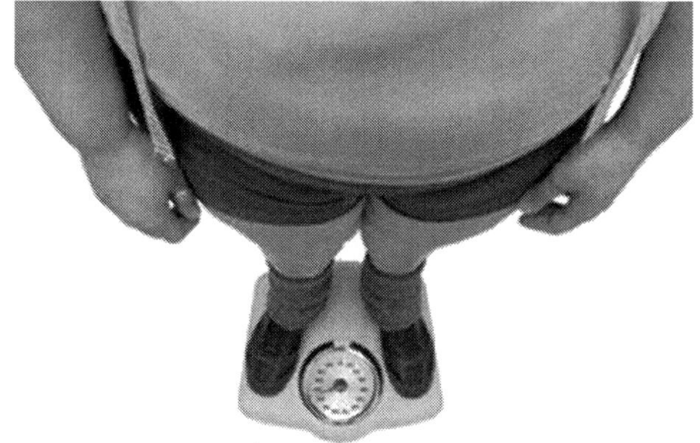

Another important health problem related to weight is obesity, defined as "a body mass index (BMI) that is equal to or greater than the 95th percentile of the age and gender specific charts developed by the Centers for Disease Control and Prevention (CDC)" (Marshall, 2013).[113] See the following BMI chart to help figure out if you are a healthy weight for your height. In general, the higher the number, the more body fat a person has.

BMI Categories: [114]

- Underweight = <18.5
- Normal weight = 18.5–24.9

- Overweight = 25–29.9
- Obesity = BMI of 30 or greater

Body Mass Index (BMI) Table for Adult Men & Women

Height (in feet and inches) / Weight (in pounds)

	Healthy Weight						Over Healthy Weight					Obese	
BMI	19	20	21	22	23	24	25	26	27	28	29	30	35
4'10"	91	96	100	105	110	115	119	124	129	134	138	143	167
4'11"	94	99	104	109	114	119	124	128	133	138	143	148	173
5'	97	102	107	112	118	123	128	133	138	143	148	153	179
5'1"	100	106	111	116	122	127	132	137	143	148	153	158	185
5'2"	104	109	115	120	126	131	136	142	147	153	158	164	191
5'3"	107	113	118	124	130	135	141	146	152	158	163	169	197
5'4"	110	116	122	128	134	140	145	151	157	163	169	174	204
5'5"	114	120	126	132	138	144	150	156	162	168	174	180	210
5'6"	118	124	130	136	142	148	155	161	167	173	179	186	216
5'7"	121	127	134	140	146	153	159	166	172	178	185	191	223
5'8"	125	131	138	144	151	158	164	171	177	184	190	197	230
5'9"	128	135	142	149	155	162	169	176	182	189	196	203	236
5'10'	132	139	146	153	160	167	174	181	188	195	202	207	243
5'11"	136	143	150	157	165	172	179	186	193	200	208	215	250
6'	140	147	154	162	169	177	184	191	199	206	213	221	258
6'1"	144	151	159	166	174	182	189	197	204	212	219	227	265
6'2"	148	155	163	171	179	186	194	202	210	218	225	233	272
6'3"	152	160	168	176	184	192	200	208	216	224	232	240	279
6'4"	156	164	172	180	189	197	205	213	221	230	238	246	287

Young adults who are obese are at higher risk for developing several other medical problems, including adult onset diabetes and cardiac disease.[115] Obese individuals are also at greater risk for developing bone and joint problems, sleep disorders, social isolation and poor body image.[116] The establishment of healthy lifestyle habits, including eating a healthy diet and becoming more physically active, are the most important steps in fighting obesity. If you are concerned about your weight or have questions about your body mass index, you should visit the student health services on your campus and speak to a medical professional. This person will be able to advise you as to the steps you can take to improve your diet, add an exercise regimen to your schedule and/or address any underlying psychological issues which may exist.

CONCLUSION

Eating disorders arise from a combination of social, cultural, psychological and genetic issues, and regardless of race, gender or sexual orientation, you are at risk.[117] If you suspect you or someone you know may have an eating disorder, contact your office of health services right away.

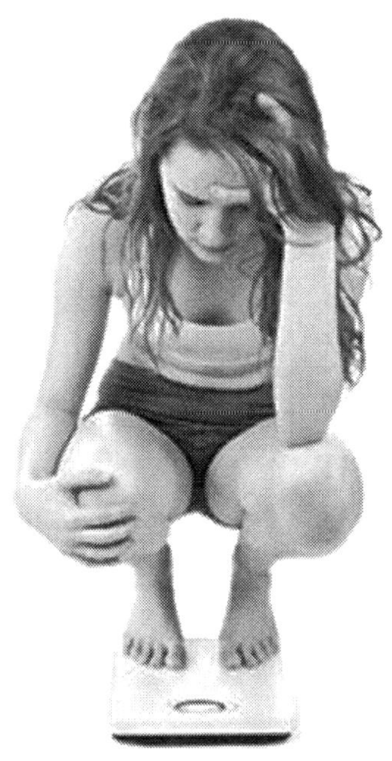

For additional information on the topics discussed in this chapter, see the Q&A section on page 64 and the resources below:

http://www.anad.org/news/the-hidden-health-crisis-on-campus-eating-disorders/

http://www.womenshealth.gov/body-image/eating-disorders/

http://www.nationaleatingdisorders.org/general-information

http://www.cdc.gov/nccdphp/dch/programs/CommunitiesPuttingPreventiontoWork/resources/obesity.htm

Mental Health

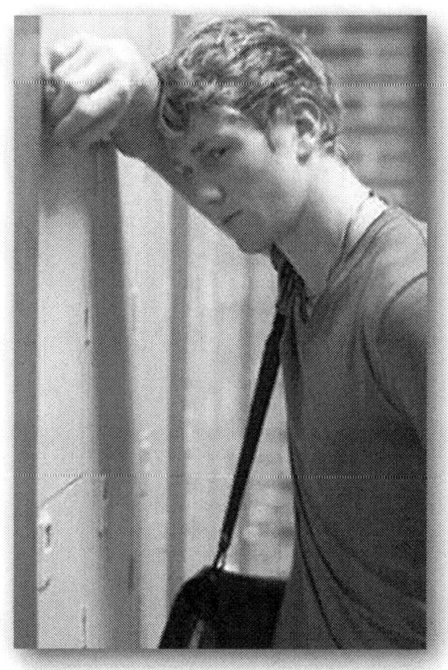

Depression and anxiety are common problems on college campuses nationwide and research shows that the average age at which these disorders surface is between 18 and 24.[118] College life can present many challenges for students, including being away from home for the first time, meeting new people, exposure to different cultures, living with new roommates and academic pressure. Because of these unique stresses, many experience symptoms of depression and/or anxiety for the first time during their college years.

DEPRESSION

Everyone feels sad from time to time, but clinical depression is another thing altogether. Depression is characterized by disturbances in mood, energy, sleep, appetite, interest and libido.[119] It affects one's ability to function, and can prevent one from experiencing joy or pleasure. People suffering from depression often have feelings of hopelessness, and sometimes even suicidal thoughts. Of course, anyone can feel sad or without hope from time to time and depression can occur as a normal response to the usual ups and downs of life. By contrast, the signs and symptoms of depression persist for longer than two weeks and interfere with one's daily life. You should seek professional help if you suffer from five or more of the symptoms listed below:[120]

- If you feel sad, empty, or hopeless;
- If you have lost interest in things you once enjoyed;
- If you have feelings of guilt or remorse for no reason;
- If you are not able to make good sound decisions;
- If you are unable to concentrate;
- If you have become increasingly fatigued or have decreased energy levels;
- If you are either unable to sleep or are sleeping too much;
- If you feel moody, irritable or agitated; and/or
- If you have thoughts about dying and suicide.

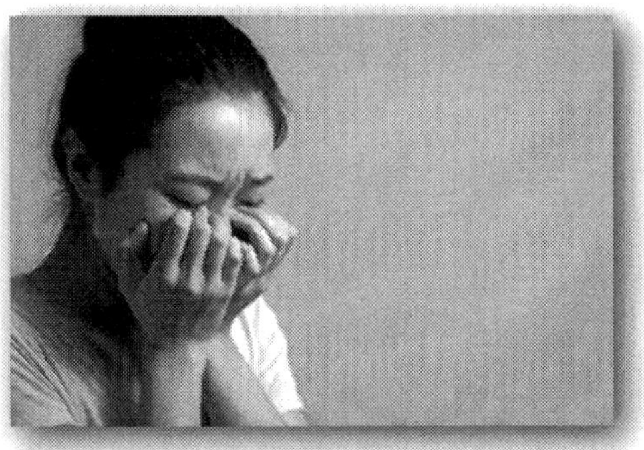

ANXIETY

Anxiety can be a common response to trouble or potential danger, and some level of anxiety is healthy and normal. However, when one's anxiety gets out of control and starts to interfere with daily living, it is important to seek professional help. Some of the symptoms that warrant professional attention are listed below:[121]

- If you worry constantly about awful things that may happen to you now or in the future;
- If you worry about things that have already happened to you;
- If you are scared and find it hard to focus on anything else;
- If you experience physical symptoms, such as heart palpitations, difficulty breathing, muscle aches, pains and headache;
- If you find it difficult to focus or concentrate, and are easily distracted;
- If you are nervous or agitated for no apparent reason;
- If you have difficulty being around people, or social situations make you uncomfortable;
- If you experience panic attacks, characterized by an increase in fear and anxiety with physical symptoms of heart palpitations and difficulty breathing.

In addition to seeking professional help to manage your anxiety, there are some other relaxation techniques that some find helpful. Among these are:

- Breathing exercises
- Yoga classes
- Simple meditation or listening to relaxing music
- Guided meditation or visual imagery
- Deep muscle relaxation exercises

CONCLUSION

The way we live our lives has a direct impact on our emotional well-being. In addition to recognizing your limits and monitoring the stressors in your life, be sure to eat a healthy diet, exercise, get plenty of rest, and avoid excessive consumption of alcoholic beverages. If you are experiencing symptoms of depression or anxiety, you are not alone. Do not wait to inform either your primary care provider or campus health professional, who will assist you in accessing counseling and other available resources.

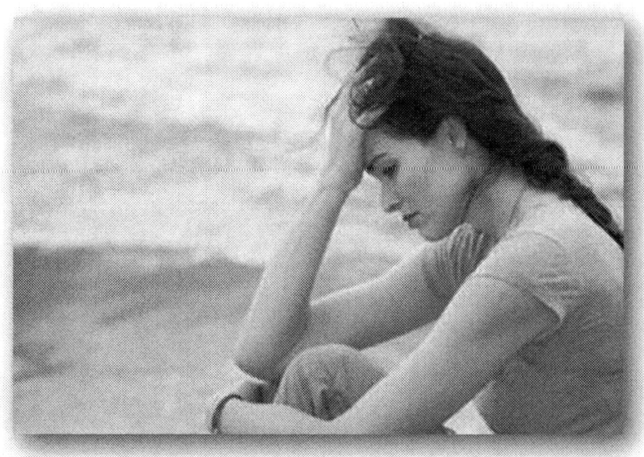

For additional information on the topics discussed in this chapter, see the Q&A section on page 64 and the resources below:

http://www.cdc.gov/mentalhealth/

http://www.cdc.gov/ViolencePrevention/suicide/index.html

http://www.cdc.gov/violenceprevention/pub/coping_with_stress_tips.html

http://www.nimh.nih.gov/health/publications/anxiety-disorders/index.shtml

http://www.nlm.nih.gov/medlineplus/depression.html

Sleep

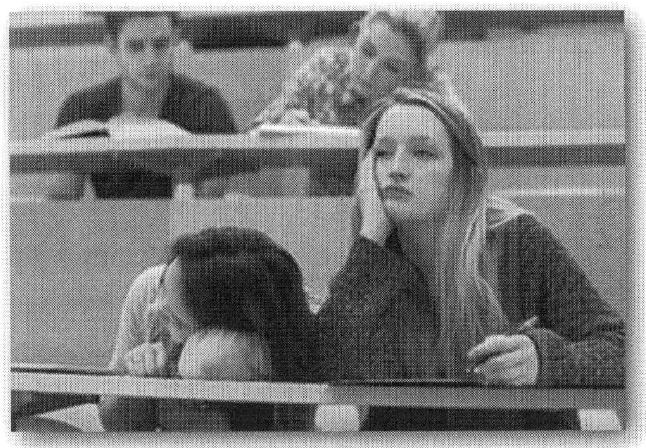

Research shows college students today sleep approximately six hours or less per night and are considered one of the most sleep-deprived populations.[122, 123] Sleeping the recommended 8 hours per night can restore body function and help to boost your immune system. Sleep also maintains your circadian rhythm (your "internal body clock," a 24-hour cycle that restores and rejuvenates your mind and body)[124] and has been shown to be an active and dynamic process that is extremely important for the maintenance of healthy motor and cognitive function.[125] Sleep deprivation, on the other hand, can lead to decreased academic performance by negatively effecting one's learning, memory, speed of processing and ability to organize one's thoughts. Sleep deprivation can also increase the risk of illness, anxiety and depression[126].

Most adults need between eight and ten hours of sleep per night, although this number may vary from person to person. Research suggests that the establishment and maintenance of a "sleep ritual," or routine that helps relax the mind and body at the end of the day can help individuals develop healthier sleep habits.

Below are tips to help establish your own sleep ritual:[127, 128]

- Establish a regular routine at bedtime. When possible, you should begin to slow down about an hour before sleep.
- As much as possible, try to go to bed at the same time each night, and get up at the same time each morning.
- Turn off electronic devices. Research shows that the blue light emitted from screens can disturb sleep patterns.[129]
- Minimize your intake of caffeine in the evening.
- Avoid drinking alcohol and/or eating a large meal before bed. If you must snack in the evening, eat foods that will help you sleep, such as peanut butter, turkey, low-fat yogurt, a banana, walnuts or almonds.
- You can also take natural sleep aids such as tryptophan, melatonin and herbal teas. Tryptophan is an essential amino acid and is found in most dairy products and protein-containing foods including cheddar cheese, low fat mozzarella, soy beans, tofu, tempeh, pumpkin and squash seeds, almonds, cashews and pistachios.[130] Melatonin is a hormone naturally found in the body which helps regulate sleep. Melatonin supplement can be found in pharmacies or most grocery stores, and the typical dose for insomnia is 0.3 - 5 mg 90 minutes before bedtime.[131] Herbal teas that are promoted for their relaxing effects include chamomile, valerian, peppermint, lavender and lemon balm.[132] There is no scientific research proving the effectiveness of these herbal teas, however, many people find them calming and effective. [133]

CONCLUSION

Sleep is vital to mind-body health, and eight hours is considered the ideal amount per night. Lack of sleep can be caused by many things, including stress, anxiety, depression, alcohol and/or a decreased level of melatonin.

It is important to maintain a healthy sleeping pattern, eat healthy and exercise daily. You should also avoid caffeinated beverages and foods after noontime. Soy nuts are a great snack any time of the day because they increase the body's level of melatonin production. It is important that you make your surroundings as relaxing as possible, removing distractions such as the television or radio and keeping the room temperature comfortable.

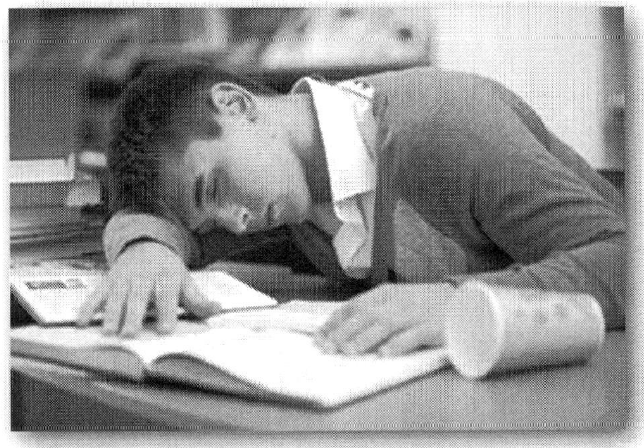

For additional information on the topics discussed in this chapter, see the Q&A section on page 64 and the resources below:

http://www.cdc.gov/features/sleep/

http://sleepfoundation.org/

Mind-Body Health

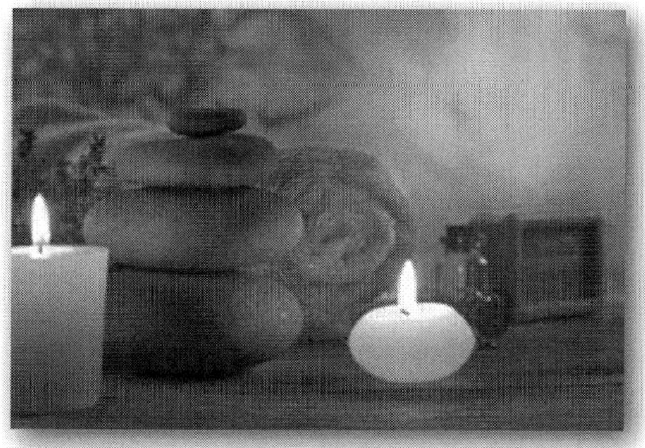

Mind-body health refers to the direct relationship between a person's physical health and their state of mind. The body responds to the way we think, feel and act and poor emotional health can harm the body's immune system, making it more susceptible to the common cold, flu or other viral and bacterial infections. Also, anxiety, depression and/or stress may contribute to poor eating habits, less exercise and decreased sleep.

Here are some helpful tips to help you take care of yourself, mind and body:[134]

Eat healthy

- Choose organic products when possible (remember, chemicals in your food become chemicals in your body).
- Eat lots of fruits, vegetables, whole grains, and nuts and minimize your intake of white flour and white sugar.
- When possible, use fresh and natural dressings, condiments and seasonings.

- When your schedule permits, try to eat three healthy meals a day with healthy snacks in between.
- It is also a good idea to remain well hydrated. Health professionals recommend that you drink 8 glasses of water per day.

Make sure you get enough sleep as sleep is vital to mind-body health. Too many students suffer from a lack of sleep, whether due to stress, a heavy course load, social activities, or for any number of other reasons. In order to maintain a healthy sleeping pattern, it is helpful if you are able to eat a healthy diet and get some strenuous exercise on a regular basis. If you are especially sensitive to caffeine, you should avoid caffeinated beverages and foods in the afternoon.

Daily exercise is useful for controlling your weight and decreasing your risk of heart disease, diabetes and cancer, among other conditions. It is also helpful in reducing anxiety, depression and insomnia.

Meditation, yoga and breath therapy are self-healing techniques that are easy to do.

- Daily meditation for five to 15 minutes will begin your day mindfully. When meditating, you should sit in a comfortable position, concentrate, relax and breathe softly and slowly.
- Yoga is a physical discipline that originated in India over 6,000 years ago. It includes breathing and relaxation techniques and is effective for alleviating muscle tension, joint problems, chronic pain, nervousness, anxiety and sleep disorders.[135]
- Breath therapy is useful for stress, anxiety, fatigue, joint pain and sleep. Its goal is to promote rhythmic breathing that makes conscious use of the muscles of the abdomen and diaphragm.[136] It involves lying on the floor, with your calves resting on a stool or chair and a weight placed on your abdomen (books for example). The practitioner breathes deeply and calmly, periodically decreasing the weight.

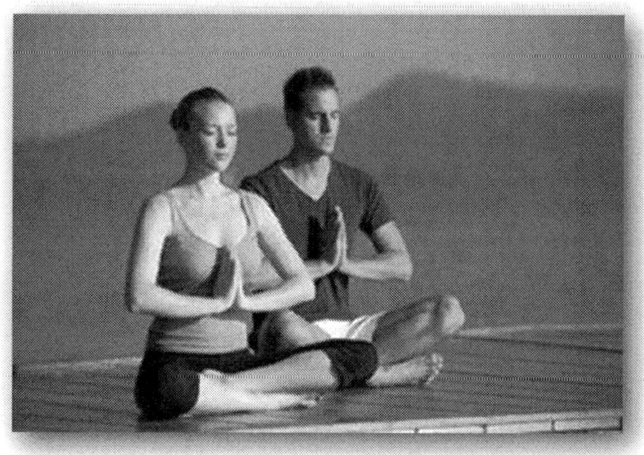

CONCLUSION

If you are experiencing increased stress, anxiety or depression, do not hesitate to inform either your healthcare provider or campus health professional. Healthy life style and self-healing therapies, and in some cases medication can help you regain your peace of mind.

Complementary and Alternative Therapies (CAM)

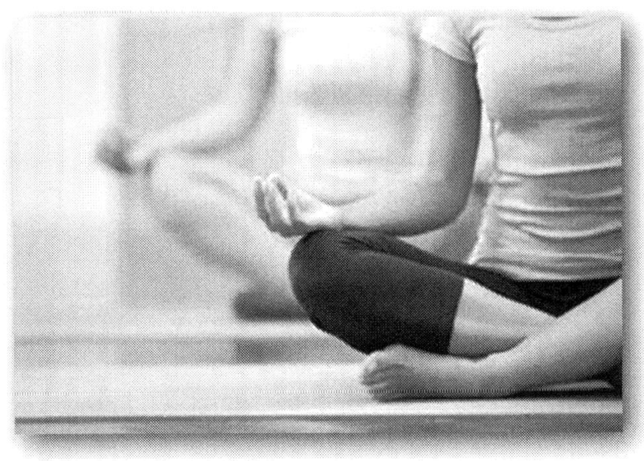

Complementary and alternative medicine (CAM) is more popular now than ever, and healthcare providers in various settings are embracing the idea of integrated medicine and incorporating CAM therapies into their practices. According to the National Center for Complementary and Alternative Therapies (NCCAM), "Complementary generally refers to using a non-mainstream approach together with conventional medicine... whereas Alternative refers to using a non-mainstream approach in place of conventional medicine."[137]

If you are interested in exploring CAM therapies, there are several options available. NCCAM breaks CAM into two categories: mind-body practices and natural products which comprise most of the CAM therapies.[138]

According to NCCAM, the most commonly used mind body CAM therapies in the United States are those listed below.[139]

Practitioners of **acupuncture** stimulate specific points on the body by inserting very thin, disposable needles into several areas of the patient's skin at defined points. This therapy is used to treat pain and cure disease.

Massage therapy is the therapeutic manipulation of the soft tissues of the body, causing the muscles to relax. There are several types of massage therapy including Swedish massage, Deep Tissue massage, Hot Stone massage, Aromatherapy, Shiatsu, Thai and Reflexology.[140]

Meditation involves quieting the mind and increasing awareness of the present moment in order to promote relaxation and stress reduction.

Movement therapies include a wide variety of approaches. Some of the more common examples include the following:

- **Alexander Technique** focuses on posture and body movement. It is used to help promote pain relief and other physical benefits.
- **The Feldenkrais Method** is a form of therapy that helps improve coordination and flexibility.
- **Hypnotherapy** refers to a patient being put into a trance, using various techniques of relaxation and guided imagery.
- **Pilates** is a series of exercises which use special equipment to help strengthen and control muscles and improve posture.
- **Reiki** is a Japanese massage therapy which attempts to focus the body's healing energies on areas of stress and/or pain.
- **Relaxation techniques** such as breathing exercises, guided imagery, and progressive muscle relaxation, are used to stimulate the body's natural relaxation response.
- **Spinal manipulation** plays an important role in physical therapy, chiropractic, osteopathic and naturopathic medicine. Spinal manipulation should only be performed by licensed healthcare professionals.

- ***Tai Chi*** and ***Qigong*** are traditional systems of Chinese exercise that combine movement and/or postures, breathing and concentration to provide physical and mental benefits to the practitioner.
- **Yoga** is an ancient South Asian system that combines physical postures or movement, breathing techniques and meditation. It is often used to address issues of balance, posture and flexibility, as well as promoting spiritual balance and focus.

Biologically based practices involve supplements including probiotics, vitamins and minerals and herbal remedies such as plants, herbs or extracts. NCCAM also identifies several other approaches that do not fall under the mind-body practices or the biologically based practices. These include **Ayurvedic Medicine** originating in India, **Traditional Chinese Medicine (TCM)**, **Homeopathy** and **Naturopathy**.[141]

While some of these complementary approaches are supported by scientific research, many have not yet been studied. Research continues and we are seeing more studies being financially supported to establish the evidence base necessary for integration and acceptance by the medical community.[142]

CONCLUSION

Before starting any new therapy, discuss the possible risks and desired benefits of the therapy you are considering with your healthcare provider. This is especially important if you are taking any prescribed medications or undergoing any specific treatments, as some of the CAM practices have been known to interfere with the effectiveness of the more traditional methods.[143]

CAM therapy's main focus is to relax the mind and reduce stress. According to Natural Medicine and Rehabilitation Journal (NMRJ), studies have shown a biochemical link between the body and the brain and the effects positive emotions have on maintaining health and wellness.[144]

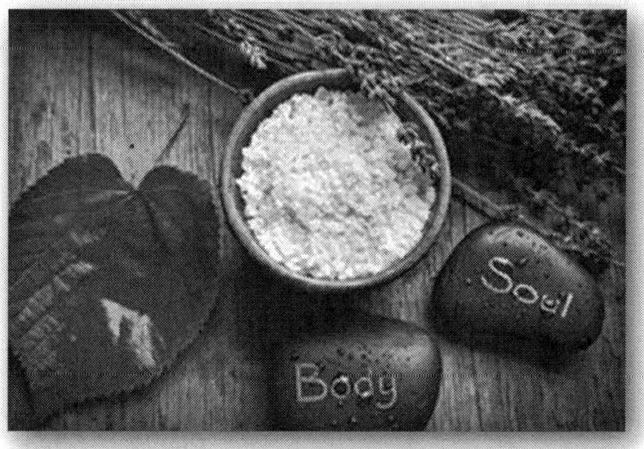

For additional information on the topics discussed in this chapter, see the Q&A section on page 64 and the resource below:

http://nccam.nih.gov/

Preventative Health

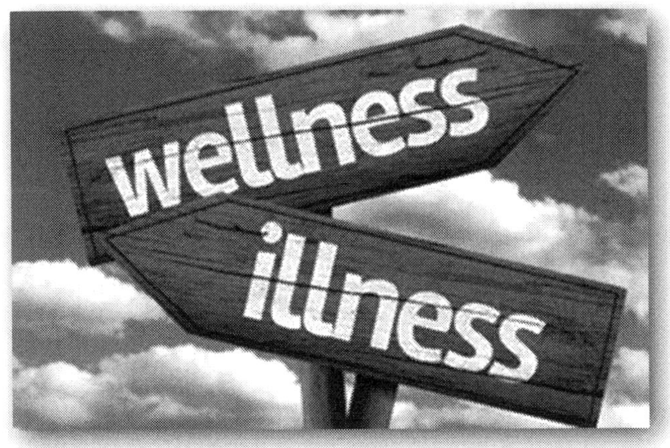

Preventative Health Tips

- *Keep immunizations current*
- *Regular physical exams*
- *Routine screenings*
- *ALWAYS wear seatbelts*
- *Use sun screen of SPF 30 >*

The most important part of preventative healthcare is the maintenance of a healthy lifestyle, including a healthy diet, daily exercise, and sufficient rest. Maintaining your health and well-being will decrease the risk of disease, disability and even death.[145] When necessary, it is also vitally important that you continue the regular treatment of any ongoing health conditions which you may already have.

Once on campus, familiarize yourself with the services offered at your college's health center. College healthcare providers are dedicated to serving students, including providing treatment for acute or chronic medical conditions. Your health services center can also provide you with information regarding preventative health strategies. The exams and screenings listed below will prove valuable in helping you to prevent or minimize disease.

Each state requires students to receive immunizations before entering college. Required immunizations may include:[146]

• Tetanus, Diphtheria, Pertussis (every 10 years) • Tdap • Measles, Mumps, Rubella • Varicella	• Influenza • Meningococcal • Hepatitis A • Hepatitis B

Screening - Maintaining a healthy lifestyle is an important part to staying healthy. However, you will need regular tests and screenings to maintain your health and feel your optimal best. See chart for the recommended health exams and screenings:[147]

Health Exams and Screenings for Women:	**Health Exams and Screenings for Men:**
• Weight, Waist Measurement and BMI – *Annually • Blood Pressure Check – *every 1-2 years • Pelvic Exam/Pap Test – *Age 21 and every 3 years thereafter • Breast Exam –* Age 20 and every 3 years thereafter • Self-Breast Exam – *Age 20 and every month thereafter • Dental – *twice yearly • Sexually transmitted infections – *Per risk • Vision Screening – *Age 20-40 • Glaucoma –*Age 40 • Hearing – *Age 18 and every 10 years thereafter • Depression Screening – *Per risk • Skin Exam – *Every 1-3 years • Cholesterol/Lipid Panel – *Every 5 years • Vaccines including HPV Vaccine	• Weight, Waist Measurement and BMI – *Annually • Blood Pressure Check – *every 1-2 years • Dental – *twice yearly • Sexually transmitted infections – *Per risk • Vision Screening/Glaucoma – *Every 2-4 years • Hearing – *Age 18 and every 10 years thereafter • Depression Screening – *Per risk • Skin Exam – *Every 1-3 years • Cholesterol/Lipid Panel – *Every 5 years • Self-Testicular Exam • Vaccines including HPV Vaccine

*Consult with your primary care provider, who may have specific recommendations based on your age, health and medical history.

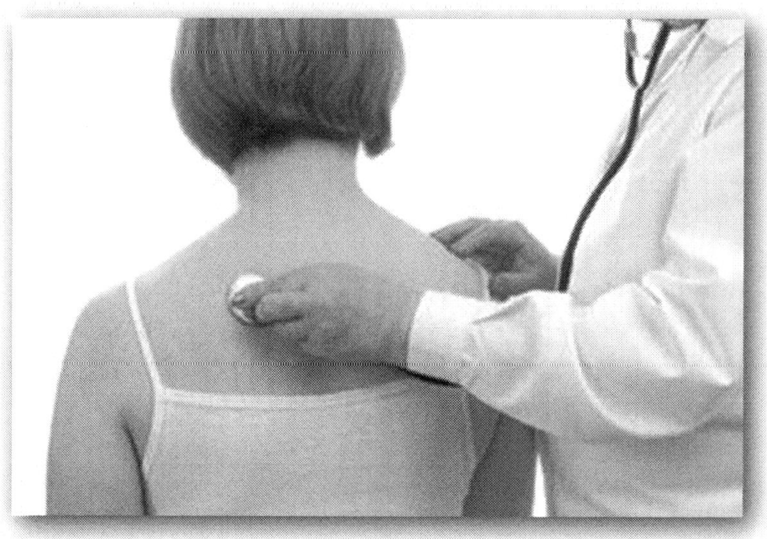

Be sure to keep track of your health information, lab tests, procedures, and any other medical care you have received. If you have been diagnosed with a medical condition, keep track of the dates of office visits and therapies, as well as any other pertinent data so that you will have it available to you should any questions arise. You should also keep a log of any medications you are taking, including the dose, name and contact information of the prescribing provider and any drug allergies and reactions.

CONCLUSION

Preventive health includes such elements as lifestyle changes, immunizations, physical examinations, screening tests and other important actions to stay healthy.[148] Preventative health is vital and should be integrated into all aspects of our daily living, including home, work, learning and social environments. [149]

According to the CDC and US Preventative Medicine, recommendations to reduce the risk of disease, illness or injury include the primary prevention examples listed:[150, 151]

- Do not smoke
- Avoid drug use and excessive alcohol use
- Maintain reproductive and sexual health
- Keep a healthy weight
- Consume a healthy diet full of fresh fruits, vegetables and whole grains
- Stay active and exercise regularly
- Preserve mental and emotional well-being
- Live injury and violence-free
- Avoid direct sun and use sunscreen
- Wear your seat belt

Focusing efforts on preventing disease, illness or injury before they occur creates a healthier environment and aids individuals in living longer, healthier, productive lives. With better health, college students will perform better in in all aspects of their lives including academics, sports, relationships and activities. You have the power to make healthy choices that will positively impact your life.

Dear Dianna Q&A

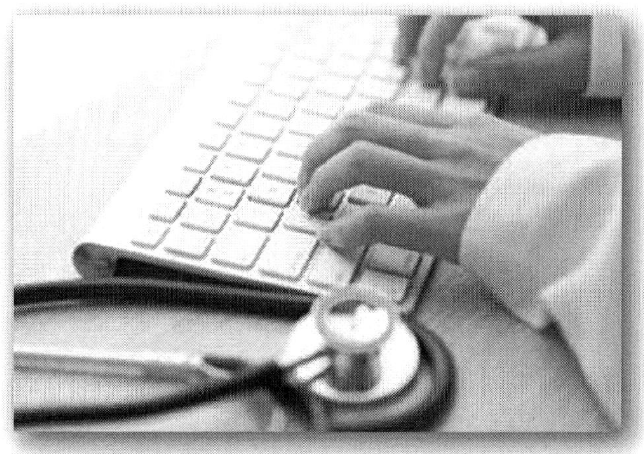

Dear Dianna,
I smoke about five or six cigarettes per week, when I am out with friends at a bar or party. Is that amount dangerous and will it affect my health?
Anonymous

Dear Anonymous,
Yes, smoking any amount is dangerous. According to the American Cardiology Association, "people who smoke less than a pack a week seem to have just as much blood vessel damage as those who smoke a pack a day or more."[152] Tobacco smoke contains roughly 4,000 chemicals, many of which are poisonous and/or carcinogenic.[153] Some of the worst of these toxins include nicotine, methane, arsenic, ammonia, formaldehyde, butane, carbon monoxide and hydrogen cyanide.[154] Smoking tobacco increases your chances of developing cancer, and also greatly increases your risk of having

a heart attack or stroke.[155] For assistance in quitting smoking, contact your college's office of health services or check out the resources below:

http://www.cdc.gov/TOBACCO/

http://www.cdc.gov/tobacco/data_statistics/fact_sheets/cessation/quitting/

http://smokefree.gov/

Dear Dianna,
I just turned 19 years old and was wondering when I should have my first pap smear?
Concerned Student

Dear Concerned Student,
The new screening recommendations advise that you receive your first pap smear at age 21, regardless whether or not you are sexually active. A pap smear can detect cancerous or precancerous conditions of the cervix. If your first pap smear is normal, then you need to repeat the process every three years.[156] However, if you experience any symptoms, or believe that you may have been exposed to an STD, you should see a healthcare professional right away.

Dear Dianna,
What can I do for my PMS? I feel awful physically, and I am so irritable one week before my period.
K.B.

Dear K.B.,
PMS can cause many symptoms including depression, anxiety, irritability, tenderness of the breasts, headache and abdominal bloating. No one knows for sure, but PMS appears to be associated with changing hormone levels during the menstrual cycle. There is no cure for PMS, but eating a healthy diet and exercising regularly may help. According to the American Academy of Family Physicians, here are some helpful tips on controlling PMS:[157]

- Eat complex carbohydrates (ie: whole grain breads, pasta and cereals), fiber and protein. Decrease your intake of sugar and fat.
- Avoid salt for a few days before your period to reduce bloating and fluid retention.
- Decrease caffeine intake. This will ease breast tenderness and tension.
- Avoid alcohol to reduce your risk of depression.
- Instead of three larger meals, eat six small meals per day.
- Be sure to exercise daily. Try to work out for 30 minutes, four to six times per week.
- Sleep eight hours per night.
- Try to avoid stressful situations until after your period.

Dear Dianna,
I had unprotected sex two weeks ago and I am worried about STDs. Should I be tested?
R.C.

Dear R.C.,
Yes, you should be evaluated and screened for STDs. If you are sexually active you are at risk. Often individuals do not experience any symptoms with STDs and can still be infected, passing it along to other partners. It is important that you be tested by a healthcare provider, and if you are infected, be sure to inform your partner so he or she can be treated as well. For more information about STDs, visit your college's office of health services or check out the resource below:

http://www.cdc.gov/STD/

Dear Dianna,
I was diagnosed with Migraine headaches by a neurologist three years ago and suffer terribly every month right before my period. Why are they so painful, and are there any alternative therapies I can use along with my prescription medication?
Kate

Dear Kate,
The cause of migraine headaches is unknown. Before a migraine presents, the arteries supplying the brain with oxygen contract, and the blood vessels then expand, causing increased pressure and leading to intense pain. Migraines can be triggered by hormonal changes, stress, alcohol consumption and foods such as chocolate, cheese, MSG and caffeine. Along with watching for triggers and taking your prescribed medication, alternative therapies exist which may offer some relief. According to the Mayo Clinic these include:[158, 159]

- Relaxation exercises such as yoga, meditation and biofeedback can both help with stress and reduce the severity and frequency of migraines.
- Acupuncture works by unblocking the blockage in particular meridians.[160] A licensed practitioner inserts very thin, disposable needles into several areas of your skin at defined points.
- Massage therapy has been shown to help reduce the frequency of migraines.

Dear Dianna,
I am a college athlete and a vegetarian. Can you give me advice on what foods I could add to my diet to increase my protein intake?
Sue K.

Dear Sue,
Protein is indeed an important nutrient that helps maintain healthy skin, bones, muscles and organs.[161] Foods high in protein include dairy products, eggs, whole grains, nuts, seeds, beans, lentils, soy products and meat substitutes. Other high protein foods to add to your meals include quinoa, buckwheat, chia, rice and beans, hummus and peanut butter.[162] It is also important for you to eat a variety of foods including fruits and vegetables. Be sure that your protein sources are low in fat and limit foods that are high in sugar, fat and salt. For more

information on vegetarian diet and healthy vegetarian food options see resources below:

http://www.vrg.org/
http://www.webmd.com/diet/ss/slideshow-vegetarian-diet
http://www.fruitsandveggiesmorematters.org/cdc-resources
http://www.vrg.org/

Dear Dianna,
I am a 22 year old male student athlete. My father has high blood pressure, and my grandfather died of a heart attack at age 45. What can I do now to prevent heart disease?
B.H.

Dear B.H.,
Because of your family history, I recommend that you have a cardiovascular disease risk assessment screening. This includes measurement of your blood pressure, body mass index, pulse and cholesterol levels.[163] I would also encourage healthy lifestyle choices, including adopting a healthy diet with no added salt, regular exercise, maintaining a healthy weight, avoiding smoking, limiting caffeine and alcohol intake and managing your stress and anxiety in a healthy way. Of course, you should also be sure to have routine check-ups, as recommended.

Dear Dianna,
Can I get a sexually transmitted disease from oral sex?
Anonymous

Dear Anonymous,
Yes indeed. It is a common misconception that you cannot contract an STD by either giving or receiving oral sex. Unprotected oral sex puts you at risk for contracting diseases such as HIV, herpes, HPV, gonorrhea, chlamydia and syphilis.[164] If you have been involved in any sexual activity

including oral sex, you should schedule an appointment at your college's office of health services to be screened for STDs. For more information on STDs see the resources below:

http://www.cdc.gov/STD/

http://www.webmd.com/sex-relationships/features/4-things-you-didnt-know-about-oral-sex

Dear Dianna,
What are the dangerous side effects of caffeine? I drink about six cups of coffee a day and sometimes more during exams.
S.K.

Dear S.K.,
According to the Mayo Clinic a healthy amount of caffeine is 200 to 300 mg per day, which is equal to about two to four cups of brewed coffee.[165] If you drink more than four cups of caffeinated coffee per day, you may experience some unpleasant side effects such as insomnia, restlessness, anxiety and irritability. In addition, research shows that caffeine use has been associated with stomach ulcers, muscle tremors, headaches and irregular heartbeat.[166] Most often, caffeine does not pose a problem for healthy individuals. However, if you experience any of the unpleasant side effects, it may be time to decrease your caffeine intake.

Dear Dianna,
Can you please explain BMI and what it means?
Thank you,
L.J.

Dear L.J.,
The BMI (Body Mass Index) is a simple statistical measurement, which tells healthcare providers whether or not a patient is at a healthy body weight relative to his/her height. The measurement does not calculate the

percentage of body fat. See the chart below to measure your BMI.[167] If you have questions or would like more information about BMI and healthy weight, you should visit your college's office of health services.

BMI Categories: [168]

- Underweight = <18.5
- Normal weight = 18.5–24.9
- Overweight = 25–29.9
- Obesity = BMI of 30 or greater

Body Mass Index (BMI) Table for Adult Men & Women

	Healthy Weight						Over Healthy Weight					Obese	
BMI	19	20	21	22	23	24	25	26	27	28	29	30	35
4'10"	91	96	100	105	110	115	119	124	129	134	138	143	167
4'11"	94	99	104	109	114	119	124	128	133	138	143	148	173
5'	97	102	107	112	118	123	128	133	138	143	148	153	179
5'1"	100	106	111	116	122	127	132	137	143	148	153	158	185
5'2"	104	109	115	120	126	131	136	142	147	153	158	164	191
5'3"	107	113	118	124	130	135	141	146	152	158	163	169	197
5'4"	110	116	122	128	134	140	145	151	157	163	169	174	204
5'5"	114	120	126	132	138	144	150	156	162	168	174	180	210
5'6"	118	124	130	136	142	148	155	161	167	173	179	186	216
5'7"	121	127	134	140	146	153	159	166	172	178	185	191	223
5'8"	125	131	138	144	151	158	164	171	177	184	190	197	230
5'9"	128	135	142	149	155	162	169	176	182	189	196	203	236
5'10'	132	139	146	153	160	167	174	181	188	195	202	207	243
5'11"	136	143	150	157	165	172	179	186	193	200	208	215	250
6'	140	147	154	162	169	177	184	191	199	206	213	221	258
6'1"	144	151	159	166	174	182	189	197	204	212	219	227	265
6'2"	148	155	163	171	179	186	194	202	210	218	225	233	272
6'3"	152	160	168	176	184	192	200	208	216	224	232	240	279
6'4"	156	164	172	180	189	197	205	213	221	230	238	246	287

Height (in feet and inches)

Weight (in pounds)

Dear Dianna,
What does SPF stand for and what number sunscreen do you recommend?
Sue F.

Dear Sue,
Sunscreens are rated with a sun protection factor (SPF) that measures a sunscreen's ability to block the sun's damaging rays (UVA/UVB). According

to the American Academy of Dermatology, sunscreen should be used every day if you are going to be exposed to the sun for longer than 20 minutes.[169] The recommendation is SPF 30 or higher. It is important to apply the sunscreen 15-20 minutes before sun exposure.

Here are some helpful tips courtesy of the American Academy of Dermatology (2015):[170]

- Generously apply sunscreen to all exposed skin using a Sun Protection Factor (SPF) of 30 or greater that provides broad-spectrum protection from both ultraviolet A (UVA) and ultraviolet B (UVB) rays. Re-apply every two hours, even on cloudy days, and after swimming or sweating.
- Wear protective clothing, such as a long-sleeved shirt, pants, a wide-brimmed hat and sunglasses, when possible.
- Seek shade when appropriate, remembering that the sun's rays are strongest between 10 a.m. and 4 p.m.
- Use extra caution near water, snow and sand as they reflect the damaging rays of the sun, which can increase your chance of sunburn.
- Get vitamin D safely through a healthy diet that includes vitamin supplements. Don't rely on the sun as a source.
- Avoid tanning beds. Ultraviolet light from the sun and tanning beds causes skin cancer and wrinkling. If you want to look like you've been in the sun, consider using a sunless self-tanning product, but you should continue to use sunscreen along with it.

Check your birthday suit on your birthday. If you notice anything on your skin that looks like it has changed, grown in size, or bleeding, be sure to see a healthcare provider or a dermatologist. Skin cancer is treatable when caught early.

Dear Dianna,
What are the signs of skin cancer and what exactly is melanoma?
M.M.

Dear M.M.,
Here are some facts about melanoma courtesy of the American Cancer Society:[171]

- Melanoma is a skin cancer that can spread earlier and more quickly than other skin cancers.
- One out of every 50 Americans will develop melanoma in their lifetime. It is the fastest growing cancer in the U.S. and worldwide.
- Melanoma is the second most common of all cancers in men and women ages 15-29.
- Roughly 80,000 Americans are diagnosed with melanoma every year - one person every 8 minutes!
- If caught in the earliest stages, melanoma is entirely treatable, but because it spreads quickly, early detection and immediate treatment is critical.
- Melanoma often starts out as a mole and can easily be removed if caught early. However, because moles are often mistaken for beauty marks, they go unnoticed. Have a dermatologist look at anything abnormal on your skin.
- Risk factors for melanoma include fair complexion, family history, severe sunburns as a child, and the use of a tanning bed ten times a year or more before age 30.
- Tanning beds are not healthier than sitting in the sun; actually, the UVA rays used in tanning beds contain three times the amount of harmful radiation emitted by the sun. UVA rays from tanning beds penetrate deep into the skin; destroying skin fibers and damaging elasticity, and causing premature aging, wrinkles, and leathery skin.
- The best ways to lower the risk of non-melanoma skin cancers are to avoid intense sunlight for long periods of time and to use sunscreen that provides both UVA and UVB protection.

A mole or freckle that changes can be the first sign of skin cancer. Watch any mole or freckle you have for changes in shape, size and color. Be aware also of any pigmented spots appearing on your skin.[172]

According to the Skin Cancer Foundation look for the ABCDEs of skin cancer:[173]

Asymmetry – one half of the mole is different from the other half;
Border – the mole or freckle is irregularly-shaped and poorly-defined, uneven;
Color – varies from one area of the mole to another, and may include shades of black, red, blue and brown;
Diameter – the mole or freckle is larger than 6 mm as a rule (diameter of pencil eraser);
Evolving - any change in the size, shape, color, elevation of the mole or freckle, or the appearance of any new symptom, including bleeding, itching or crusting.

The best way to protect yourself is to limit your time in the sun between 10:00 a.m. and 4:00 p.m. Always wear a broad-spectrum sunscreen with a sun protection factor (SPF) of 30 or greater, and when possible, cover yourself up with a hat, sun glasses and long-sleeved shirt. Make an appointment with your healthcare provider or a dermatologist immediately if you notice anything abnormal on your skin.

Dear Dianna,
How soon after a missed period can I take a pregnancy test?
Diane

Dear Diane,
Pregnancy tests detect the hormone human chorionic gonadotropin (HCG). It is found in both urine and blood during pregnancy and can be identified as early as 10 days after conception.[174] Many home pregnancy tests can now be taken on the first day of your missed period; however, it is advised to wait one week after your missed period for more accurate

results.[175] There is also a blood test that can be taken by a healthcare provider which can detect the HCG earlier than the urine test. [176]

Dear Dianna,
I have terrible facial acne. Do you have any suggestions for treatment?
Debbie A.

Dear Debbie,
There are many treatment options that exist for acne including over the counter topical products you can purchase at the pharmacy. These agents are effective in patients with mild to moderate acne, sometimes in combination with topical antibiotics. Oral antibiotics are used with patients whose acne is moderate to severe. Interestingly, birth control pills have also been effective in treating more serious cases of acne.[177] However, the first thing you should do is see your primary care provider or schedule an appointment at your college health services. They will determine what treatment option is best for you. If you are looking for a natural way to manage your acne, research shows that applying tea tree oil to affected areas for 20 minutes per day has been shown to be safe and effective.[178, 179] Whatever treatment option you chose, be sure to avoid touching your face and try to keep your hair away from your face. Also, women should avoid heavy make-up. Keep your skin as natural as possible.

Dear Dianna,
How do I know if I have depression?
Anonymous

Dear Anonymous,
According to the National Institute of Mental Health, there are several different types of depression, and "the severity, frequency and duration of symptoms will vary depending on the individual and his or her particular illness."[180] Depression affects one's ability to function and experience joy and/or pleasure. People who suffer from depression may experience

feelings of hopelessness, sometimes even suicidal thoughts. It is very important for you to seek professional help if you suffer from five or more of the symptoms listed below for longer than a two week period:[181]

- If you feel sad, empty, or hopeless;
- If you have lost interest in things you once enjoyed;
- If you have feelings of guilt or remorse for no reason;
- If you are not able to make good sound decisions;
- If you are unable to study or concentrate;
- If you have become increasingly fatigued, or have decreased energy levels;
- If you are either unable to sleep or are sleeping too much;
- If you feel moody, irritable or agitated;
- If you have thoughts about dying or suicide.

Don't wait! You are not alone, and there are people who can help you. Contact your college's office of health services and schedule an appointment to speak with a counselor.

Dear Dianna,
Is it possible to get an STD from having sexual relations with someone of the same gender?
L.F.

Dear L.F.,
Regardless of your sexual orientation, if you are involved in a sexual relationship you are putting yourself at risk for contracting STDs. You should be screened for STDs if you are engaging in any type of sexual activities. Practicing safe sex is a must no matter what your orientation. For more information on LGBT health or STDs see the resources below:

http://www.cdc.gov/lgbthealth/youth-resources.htm

http://www.lgbthealtheducation.org/publications/lgbt-health-resources/

Dear Dianna,
Can energy drinks be dangerous?
D.J.

Dear D.J.,
Energy drinks such as Red Bull and Rock Star contain large amounts of caffeine and other stimulants such as guarana and ginseng.[182] The amount of caffeine can range anywhere from 55 milligrams to over 250 milligrams.[183] The caffeine in energy drinks can cause some very unpleasant side effects including increased heart rate, blood pressure, headaches, nervousness, decreased sleep, itching and dehydration.[184] In combination with alcohol, energy drinks can be very dangerous. In addition to dehydration, the stimulant in the energy drink can mask intoxication causing carelessness and risky behaviors.[185] Everyone responds differently to caffeine and therefore should be cautious when ingesting such products. Moderation is the key for everything including energy drinks if you choose to consume them.

Dear Dianna,
What is the difference between a cold and the flu?
M.Q.

Dear M.Q.,
A common cold and the flu may cause many of the same symptoms. However, a cold is generally mild, while the flu tends to be more severe. Those suffering from a cold often experience fatigue, sneezing, coughing and a runny nose, and may or may not have a low-grade fever. You may also have body aches, a scratchy, irritated or sore throat, a headache and watery eyes. The flu starts more abruptly, and may cause immediate feelings of weakness and fatigue. You will probably also experience a fever, dry cough, runny nose, chills, body aches, headache, eye pain, and/or a sore throat. It usually takes longer to get over the flu than it does a common cold. There

are over 100 different viruses that can cause a cold, and a lesser number of viruses that cause the flu.[185] While there are vaccines which provide some protection from the flu, there are unfortunately no medications that can cure either a cold or the flu.

Symptom	Cold	Flu
Fever	Uncommon, usually no fever or low grade, 99.0 to 100 degrees	High, 101 to 104 degrees – can last 3-4 days
Cough/Chest Discomfort	Usually hacking, mild	Common, can become severe
Sore Throat	Common	Occasionally
Fatigue	Uncommon or mild	Beginning of illness, can last up to 2 weeks
Chest Discomfort	Mild	Severe
Stuffy Nose	Common	Occasionally
Aches/Pains	Mild	Severe
Headache	Uncommon	Usually Severe

How to treat your cold or flu symptoms:[187, 188]

Rest is essential, especially while you have a fever. Drink lots of fluids! Remaining hydrated is also important if you have a fever. Fluids will also help to loosen mucus in your nose and throat, easing congestion.

To help relieve a sore throat, drink warm tea with honey and gargle with warm salt water a few times a day.

Some helpful hints for preventing seasonal flu:[189, 190]
Wash your hands frequently with warm water and soap.

When coughing or sneezing, cover your nose and mouth with a tissue to prevent the spread of the virus.

Eat three healthy meals a day and drink plenty of fluids.

Do not share food or drinks.

Exercise daily for a minimum of 30 minutes.

Avoid close contact with others who may be infected.

Get a flu shot annually.

Dear Dianna,
Can I catch a disease from getting a tattoo?
W.A.

Dear W.A.,
Tattoos are permanent ink designs drawn directly onto the skin. During the placement process the skin is breached which puts the individual at risk for skin infections and other possible conditions.[191]

According to the Mayo Clinic specific risks of tattoos include:[192]

- Blood-borne diseases such as hepatitis B and hepatitis C caused by contaminated equipment;
- Allergic reactions to the dyes causing itching and irritation;

- Skin infection causing pain, warmth, redness, swelling and discharge at the site;
- Scar tissue causing raised, hardened areas.

If you decide to get a tattoo, be sure to research the artist carefully. Remember a tattoo is permanent and you will want to be certain about your decision.

Dear Dianna,
Is hookah smoking safe?
J.H.

Dear J.H.,
According to the CDC, hookah smoking has many of the same health risks as smoking cigarettes and is not a safe alternative. In addition to the toxic agents that contribute to clogged arteries, heart disease, lung, bladder and oral cancers, hookah smokers can contract infections that may be passed by other smokers sharing a hookah. Additionally secondhand smoke from hookahs can pose health risks for nonsmokers.[193] If you are a hookah smoker or smoke cigarettes, you should quit to reduce health risks.

Dear Dianna,
Two players on my basketball team have MRSA. What is it and is it contagious?
N.D.

Dear N.D.,
MRSA stands for Methicillin-resistant Staphylococcus aureus. It is a bacterium that causes infection and it is resistant to many of the antibiotics healthcare providers regularly use to treat infections. The type of MRSA that is associated with athletes, such as your teammates, is community-associated MRSA.[194] It is transmitted by close skin to skin contact and it will

be important for your teammates to be extra careful while they are infected with this bacteria. In addition to practicing good hygiene, The National Institute of health suggests for MRSA prevention:[195]

- Keeping cuts and scrapes clean and covered with a bandage until fully healed;
- Avoiding contact with other individuals that have wounds or bandages;
- Avoiding sharing personal items, such as towels, washcloths, razors, or clothes;
- Washing soiled sheets, towels, and clothes in hot water with bleach and dry in a hot dryer.

MRSA can appear on the skin as one or more infected bumps, pimples, boils or abscesses. Be sure to see a healthcare provider if you notice any of the above. Treatment may be necessary and could include draining the infection and a course of antibiotics.

Dear Dianna,
What are the dangers of pot if I smoke it only on occasion?
Todd

Dear Todd,
In addition to respiratory issues such as daily cough, congestion and frequent lung infections, marijuana also affects brain development.[196] According to the National Institute on Drug Abuse, frequent marijuana use by young adults negatively impacts memory, learning and thinking. These effects can be long lasting and even permanent.[197] Research also suggests that marijuana use may negatively affect one's physical and emotional health, maintaining relationships, self-motivation and academic performance. "For example, marijuana use is associated with a higher likelihood of dropping out of school."[198] Studies have also shown that marijuana use during the adolescent years is also linked to depression and mental

illness.[199] Because of the harm marijuana causes, it is recommended that young adults avoid the use of marijuana all together.[200] For more information on marijuana and other drugs see the resource below:

http://www.nlm.nih.gov/learn-about-drugs.html

Conclusion

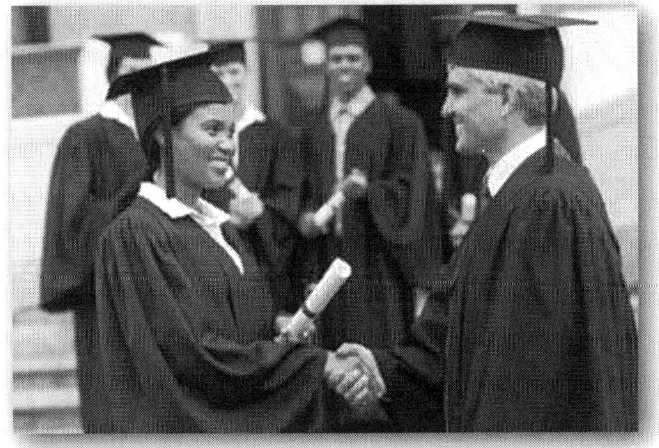

College students face many health challenges in the areas of alcohol, drugs, eating disorders, exercise, mental health, nutrition, sexuality, sleep and tobacco. Students who maintain their health during the college experience give themselves the opportunity to achieve optimal performance. Students who know the facts, adopt healthy habits and maintain a balanced lifestyle during college, will lead healthier and more productive lives.

About the Author

Dianna M. Jones, Doctor of Nursing Practice and board certified Family Nurse Practitioner, serves as the Director of Health Services at Regis College. Dianna has over fourteen years of experience treating young adults and college students.

Dianna also serves as an adjunct faculty member at Regis College in the graduate nursing program, and teaches health and wellness classes to the undergraduate population. Her work as a contributing editor has been published in textbooks, and she has been featured on radio and evening news programs.

Dianna earned her BA from Tufts University and her MS and DNP from Regis College. She lives in eastern Massachusetts with her husband and their twins.

Endnotes

1 Preamble to the Constitution of the World Health Organization as adopted by the International Health Conference, New York, 19-22 June, 1946; signed on 22 July 1946 by the representatives of 61 States (Official Records of the World Health Organization, no. 2, p. 100) and entered into force on 7 April 1948.

2 https://www.education.tas.gov.au/documentcentre/Documents/Tas-Curriculum-K-10-Health-and-Wellbeing-Syllabus-and-Support.pdf

3 The American Heritage® Dictionary of the English Language, Fourth Edition copyright ©2000 by Houghton Mifflin Company.

4 The American Heritage® Dictionary of the English Language, Fourth Edition copyright ©2000 by Houghton Mifflin Company.

5 www.wellbeingonline.wsu.edu/social

6 http://wellness.ucr.edu/spiritual_wellness.html

7 Edlin, Health & Wellness 11th ed. Jones and Bartlett: Burlington, MA

8 Edlin, Health & Wellness 11th ed. Jones and Bartlett: Burlington, MA

9 Edlin, Health & Wellness 11th ed. Jones and Bartlett: Burlington, MA

[10] http://newsroom.ucla.edu/portal/ucla/More-College-Freshmen-Committed-6754.aspx?RelNum=6754

[11] http://pubs.niaaa.nih.gov/publications/arh283/111-120.htm

[12] http://pubs.niaaa.nih.gov/publications/arh283/111-120.htm

[13] http://www.nlm.nih.gov/medlineplus/drugsandyoungpeople.html

[14] http://www.niaaa.nih.gov/alcohol-health/overview-alcohol-consumption/moderate-binge-drinking

[15] http://www.mayomedicallaboratories.com/test-catalog/Clinical+and+Interpretive/8264

[16] National Institute on Alcohol Abuse and Alcoholism (NIAAA, 2013)

[17] http://www.niaaa.nih.gov/alcohol-health/special-populations-co-occurring-disorders/college-drinking

[18] http://www.collegedrinkingprevention.gov/niaaacollegematerials/panel01/highrisk_04.aspx

[19] http://www.nationalsafetycommission.com/drivers-ed/florida-tlsae.html

[20] http://www.nationalsafetycommission.com/drivers-ed/florida-tlsae.html

[21] http://www.niaaa.nih.gov/alcohol-health/overview-alcohol-consumption/standard-drink

[22] http://pubs.niaaa.nih.gov/publications/aa46.htm

23 http://pubs.niaaa.nih.gov/publications/aa46.htm

24 http://pubs.niaaa.nih.gov/publications/aa46.htm

25 http://www.samhsa.gov/data/nsduh/2k11results/nsduhresults2011.htm#2.3

26 Haiken, (2012) http://www.forbes.com/sites/melaniehaiken/2012/06/13/spice-vs-bath-salts-the-other-designer-drug-scare/

27 http://www.cdc.gov

28 http://www.drugfreeworld.org/drugfacts/crackcocaine.html

29 http://www.stopcocaineaddiction.com/Cocaine-statistics.htm

30 http://www.willisfraternity.com/wfdata/files/conclusion.pdf

31 http://www.heroin.ws/Heroin-Effects.htm

32 University of Texas (2013) http://www.healthyhorns.utexas.edu/college druguse.html

33 Willis,(2013) http://www.willisfraternity.com/wfdata/files/conclusion.pdf

34 http://www.drugabuse.gov/publications/drugfacts/marijuana

35 Willis,(2013) http://www.willisfraternity.com/wfdata/files/conclusion.pdf

36 Willis,(2013) http://www.willisfraternity.com/wfdata/files/conclusion.pdf

37 www.emergency.com/roofies.htm

38 http://www.talkaboutrx.org/documents/GetTheFacts.pdf

39 http://www.drugabuse.gov/publications/drugfacts/stimulant-adhd-medications-methylphenidate-amphetamines

40 http://www.drugabuse.gov/publications/drugfacts/stimulant-adhd-medications-methylphenidate-amphetamines

41 http://www.acha.org/

42 http://www.mass.gov/eohhs/gov/departments/dph/programs/mtcp/

43 American Smoke Out, (2012)

44 http://www.reed.edu/health_center/drug_resources/self_assessment_resources.html

45 Mangubat (2013) http://www.theprospect.net/the-art-of-the-college-sexuality-crisis-10291

46 Sams, B. http://star.txstate.edu/node/1243

47 http://www.cdc.gov/lgbthealth/about.htm

48 Edlin & Golanty Health & Wellness 11th ed. Jones and Bartlett: Burlington, MA, pg234

49 http://goaskalice.columbia.edu/whats-std

50 Edlin & Golanty Health & Wellness 11th ed. Jones and Bartlett: Burlington, MA, pg234

51 CDC http://www.cdc.gov/condomeffectiveness/latex.htm

52 CDC http://www.cdc.gov/std/stats/sti-estimates-fact-sheet-feb-2013.pdf

53 CDC http://www.cdc.gov/nchhstp/newsroom/docs/STD-Trends-508.pdf

54 CDC http://www.cdc.gov/std/stats/sti-estimates-fact-sheet-feb-2013.pdf

55 CDC http://www.cdc.gov/std/hpv/stdfact-hpv.htm

56 STIFact-HPV vaccine.htmhttp://medscape.com/viewarticle/423555_100

57 www.cdc.gov/sd/hpv/STIFactHPVvaccine.htm

58 http://www.cdc.gov/std/HPV/STDFact-HPV-and-men.htm

59 http://www.cdc.gov/STI/chlamydia/STIFact-chlamydia.htm

60 http://www.cdc.gov/STI/gonorrhea/STIFactgonorrhea.htm

61 http://goaskalicc.columbia.edu/whats-std

62 http://goaskalice.columbia.edu/college-students-and-stis

63 http://www.cdc.gov/std/syphilis/STDFact-Syphilis-detailed.htm

64 Edlin, Health & Wellness 11th ed. Jones and Bartlett: Burlington, MA

65 http://www.cdc.gov/std/trichomonas/stdfact-trichomoniasis.htm

66 http://www.cdc.gov/std/trichomonas/stdfact-trichomoniasis.htm

67 http://www.cdc.gov/std/PID/STDFact-PID.htm

68 http://www.mayoclinic.org/diseases-conditions/pelvic-inflammatory-disease/basics/complications/CON-20022341

69 http://www.cdc.gov/hepatitis/HBV/PDFs/HepBSexualHealth.pdf

70 http://www.std411.org/testing.htm

71 http://www.ncbi.nlm.nih.gov/pubmed/19278182

72 Hamilton BE, Martin JA, Ventura SJ. Births: Preliminary data for 2009. National Vital Statistics Reports 2010;59(3).

73 National Campaign to Prevent Teen and Unplanned Pregnancy. (2007). Unplanned Pregnancy Among 20-Somethings: The FullStory. Washington, DC: Author.

74 http://abcnews.go.com/Health/cdc-40-percent-us-births-unintended/story?id=16840288

75 http://www.cdc.gov/reproductivehealth/unintendedpregnancy/contraception.htm

76 Peterson, (2013) http://newsinfo.iu.edu/tips/page/normal/3383.html

77 http://www.cdc.gov/violenceprevention/pdf/sv-datasheet-a.pdf

78 http://womenshealth.gov/publications/our-publications/fact-sheet/sexual-assault.html#b

79 Zagorsky and Smith (2011) http://www.medicalnewstoday.com/articles/236994.php

80 http://www.choosemyplate.gov/about.html

81 http://kidshealth.org/parent/nutrition_center/healthy_eating/myplate.html

[82] http://ods.od.nih.gov/factsheets/Calcium-HealthProfessional/

[83] http://ods.od.nih.gov/factsheets/Calcium-HealthProfessional/

[84] http://www.mayoclinic.com/health/fat-grams/HQ00671

[85] Purcell (2006), www.bjs.com

[86] Purcell (2006), www.bjs.com

[87] http://www.mayoclinic.org/healthy-living/nutrition-and-healthy-eating/in-depth/vegetarian-diet/art-20046446?pg=2

[88] http://www.healthaliciousness.com/articles/natural-foods-high-in-iodine.php

[89] http://www.healthaliciousness.com/articles/foods-high-in-vitamin-B12.php

[90] http://www.mayoclinic.org/healthy-living/nutrition-and-healthy-eating/in-depth/vegetarian-diet/art-20046446?pg=2

[91] http://www.mayoclinic.org/healthy-living/nutrition-and-healthy-eating/in-depth/vegetarian-diet/art-20046446

[92] http://www.webmd.com/diet/features/beans-protein-rich-superfoods

[93] http://lowcarbdiets.about.com/od/lowcarbsuperfoods/a/salmonbenefits.htm

[94] http://www.whfoods.com/genpage.php?tname=foodspice&dbid=128

[95] http://articles.mercola.com/sites/articles/archive/2013/10/28/apple-health-benefits.aspx

96 http://www.care2.com/greenliving/13-health-benefits-of-oranges.html

97 http://www.whfoods.com/genpage.php?tname=foodspice&dbid=37

98 http://www.heart.org/HEARTORG/GettingHealthy/NutritionCenter/HealthyDietGoals/Sugars-and-Carbohydrates_UCM_303296_Article.jsp

99 http://www.americanheart.org/presenter.jhtml?identifier=801

100 http://www.sciencedaily.com/articles/a/anaerobic_exercise.htm (1998-2013 Mayo Foundation for Medical Education and Research (MFMER)

101 http://kidshealth.org/teen/school_jobs/college/exercise.html#

102 http://www.mayoclinic.com/health/aerobic-exercise/EP00002/NSECTIONGROUP=2

103 Burke (2013) http://www.mensfitness.com/training/build-muscle5-ways-to-cool-down-after-a-workout

104 bodynews.com/2006_Articles/5_Super_Simple_Exercise_Tips.htm,

105 www.be-with-you.com/dew/WaterAndOurBody.html,

106 http://www.webmd.com/parenting/features/healthy-beverages

107 http://www.freedrinkingwater.com/water-education/water-health.htm

108 http://www.waldenbehavioralcare.com/resources/popular-searches/eating-disorders-among-college-students/

109 http://www.nlm.nih.gov/medlineplus/ency/article/000362.htm,

110 http://www.nationaleatingdisorders.org/anorexia-nervosa

111 http://www.nationaleatingdisorders.org

112 http://www.mayoclinic.com/health/eating-disorders/DS00294/DSECTION=symptoms

113 http://www.wikihow.com/Calculate-Your-Body-Mass-Index-(BMI) Beth Marshall, CHES, DrPH

114 http://www.cdc.gov/healthyweight/assessing/bmi/adult_bmi/

115 http://www.cdc.gov/healthyyouth/obesity/facts.htm

116 http://www.jhsph.edu/research/centers-and-institutes/center-for-adolescent-health/_includes/Obesity_Standalone.pdf

117 Smolak, L., & Striegel-Moore, R. (2001). Challenging the myth of the golden girl: Ethnicity and eating disorders. In Eating Disorders: Innovative Directions in Research and Practice. Eds. Striegel-Moore & Smolak. Published by APA, Washington, D.C.

118 http://psychcentral.com/lib/depression-and-anxiety-among-college-students/0001425?pp=2

119 http://www.cpcwa.org/InformationAndResources/misigns.html

120 http://www.nimh.nih.gov/health/publications/depression-and-college-students/index.shtml

121 http://www.nimh.nih.gov/health/publications/depression-and-college-students/index.shtml

122 http://www.uhs.uga.edu/sleep/

123 http://campusmindworks.org/students/self_care/sleep.asp

124 http://www.mayoclinic.com/health/sleep/HQ01387

125 http://www.uhs.uga.edu/sleep/

126 http://www.health.harvard.edu/newsletters/Harvard_Mental_Health_Letter/2009/July/Sleep-and-mental-health

127 http://www.sleepnet.com/tips.htm

128 http://www.helpguide.org/life/sleep_tips.htm

129 Boston Globe, January 13, 2013

130 http://www.healthaliciousness.com/articles/high-tryptophan-foods.php

131 http://www.nlm.nih.gov/medlineplus/druginfo/natural/940.html

132 http://www.brown.edu/Student_Services/Health_Services/Health_Education/common_college_health_issues/sleep.php

133 http://www.webmd.com/sleep-disorders/excessive-sleepiness-10/sleep-supplements-herbs?page=2

134 http://www.studentwellness.org/anxiety/?gclid=CKa1x53dhrYCFcXb4AoduDEAVA

135 Baptiste, B. (2002), Journey Into Power. New York: Fireside

136 Vukovic, L. (2006), The Complete Guide To Natural Healing. New York: Weider Publication

137 http://nccam.nih.gov/health/whatiscam

138 http://nccam.nih.gov/health/whatiscam#cvsa

139 http://nccam.nih.gov/health/whatiscam

140 http://altmedicine.about.com/od/massage/a/massage_types.htm

141 http://nccam.nih.gov/health/whatiscam#cvsa

142 http://nccam.nih.gov/news/camstats/2007/camsurvey_fs1.htm

143 http://nmrnj.com/

144 http://nmrnj.com/

145 http://www.mass.gov/eohhs/gov/departments/dph/programs/community-health/

146 http://www.mass.gov/eohhs/gov/departments/dph/programs/id/immunization/

147 http://www.mass.gov/eohhs/gov/departments/dph/programs/community-health/primarycare-healthaccess/school-health/school-health-screening.html

[148] https://www.marshfieldclinic.org/healthy-living/preventive-care/why-important

[149] http://www.cdc.gov/features/preventionstrategy/

[150] http://www.cdc.gov/features/preventionstrategy

[151] http://www.uspreventivemedicine.com/High-Tech-Diagnostics/Why-Preventive-Medicine.aspx

[152] American Cardiology Association (2013)

[153] http://www.osteopathic.org/osteopathic-health/about-your-health/health-conditions-library/general-health/Pages/secondhand-smoke.aspx

[154] http://www.lung.org/stop-smoking/about-smoking/facts-figures/whats-in-a-cigarette.html

[155] http://www.nhlbi.nih.gov/health/health-topics/topics/smo/

[156] ACOG (2013) http://www.acog.org/~/media/Districts/District%20II/PDFs/USPSTF_CervicalCa_Screening_Guidelines.pdf?dmc=1

[157] http://familydoctor.org/141.xml

[158] http://www.mayoclinic.org/diseases-conditions/migraine-headache/basics/alternative-medicine/CON-20026358

[159] http://www.webmd.com/balance/nontraditional-headache-treatments

[160] http://doctorliu.org/services/acupuncture/migraine?gclid=CLH5wtKl8bsCFSRk7Aodm3YAgQ

[161] http://www.mayoclinic.org/healthy-living/nutrition-and-healthy-eating/in-depth/vegetarian-diet/art-20046446?pg=2

[162] http://greatist.com/health/complete-vegetarian-proteins

[163] Nash, (2007). The Positive Line

[164] http://std.about.com/od/riskfactorsforstds/a/oralsexsafesex.htm

[165] Mayo Clinic (2013)

[166] www.Alcoholism and Drug Addiction Research Foundation.org

[167] http://healthvermont.gov/pubs/disease_control/2003/2003-02.aspx

[168] http://www.cdc.gov/healthyweight/assessing/bmi/adult_bmi/

[169] American Academy of Dermatology (2007)

[170] https://www.aad.org/media/stats/prevention-and-care/sunscreen-faqs

[171] http://www.cancer.org/cancer/skincancer-melanoma/overviewguide/melanoma-skin-cancer-overview-what-is-melanoma?sitearea=CRI

[172] http://www.aad.org/public/News DermInfo/./htm

[173] http://www.skincancer.org/skin-cancer-information/melanoma/melanoma-warning-signs-and-images/do-you-know-your-abcdes#panel1-1

[174] http://www.nlm.nih.gov/medlineplus/ency/article/003432.htm

[175] http://womenshealth.gov/publications/our-publications/fact-sheet/pregnancy-tests.html#e

[176] http://womenshealth.gov/publications/our-publications/fact-sheet/pregnancy-tests.html#e

[177] STEVEN FELDMAN, M.D., PH.D., RACHEL E. CARECCIA, M.D., KELLY L. BARHAM, M.D., and JOHN HANCOX, M.D., Wake Forest University School of Medicine, Winston-Salem, North Carolina Am Fam Physician. 2004 May 1;69(9):2123-2130.

[178] http://www.mayoclinic.org/drugs-supplements/tea-tree-oil/dosing/hrb-20060086

[179] http://www.webmd.com/skin-problems-and-treatments/acne/features/tea-tree-oil-treats-skin-problems

[180] http://www.nimh.nih.gov/index.shtml

[181] NIMH (2008) http://www.nimh.nih.gov/health/topics/depression/index.shtml?utm_content=buffera397a&utm_source=buffer&utm_medium=twitter&utm_campaign=Buffer

[182] http://www.brown.edu/Student_Services/Health_Services/Health_Education/alcohol,_tobacco,_&_other_drugs/energy_drinks.php

[183] http://www.webmd.com/food-recipes/news/20121025/how-much-caffeine-energy-drink

[184] http://www.brown.edu/Student_Services/Health_Services/Health_Education/alcohol,_tobacco,_&_other_drugs/energy_drinks.php

[185] http://www.brown.edu/Student_Services/Health_Services/Health_Education/alcohol,_tobacco,_&_other_drugs/energy_drinks.php

[186] http://www.cdc.gov/flu/about/qa/coldflu.htm

187 http://www.webmd.com/cold-and-flu/8-tips-to-treat-colds-and-flu-the-natural-way

188 http://www.cdc.gov/getsmart/antibiotic-use/uri/colds.html

189 http://www.webmd.com/cold-and-flu/8-tips-to-treat-colds-and-flu-the-natural-way

190 http://www.cdc.gov/getsmart/antibiotic-use/uri/colds.html

191 http://www.mayoclinic.org/healthy-living/adult-health/in-depth/tattoos-and-piercings/art-20045067

192 http://www.mayoclinic.org/healthy-living/adult-health/in-depth/tattoos-and-piercings/art-20045067

193 http://www.cdc.gov/tobacco/data_statistics/fact_sheets/tobacco_industry/hookahs/

194 http://www.mayoclinic.org/diseases-conditions/mrsa/basics/definition/con-20024479

195 http://www.nlm.nih.gov/medlineplus/mrsa.html

196 http://www.drugabuse.gov/publications/drugfacts/marijuana

197 http://www.drugabuse.gov/publications/drugfacts/marijuana

198 http://www.drugabuse.gov/publications/drugfacts/marijuana

199 http://www.drugabuse.gov/publications/drugfacts/marijuana

200 http://health.usnews.com/health-news/blogs/health-advice/2009/05/15/is-occasional-marijuana-use-bad-foradolescents

Photo Credits/Shutterstock.com

a) Michealjung/Shutterstock.com title page
b) Dirima/Shutterstock.com p.1
c) Diego Cervo/Shutterstock.com p.3
d) Kentoh/Shutterstock.com p.4
e) LaCameraChiara/Shutterstock.com p.5
f) Tommaso79/Shutterstock.com p.6
g) Gang Liu/Shutterstock.com p.11
h) Verkhovynets Taras/Shutterstock.com p.13
i) Rock and Wasp/Shutterstock.com p.14
j) William Perugini/Shutterstock.com p.16
k) Pressmaster/Shutterstock.com p.22
l) Brocreative/Shutterstock.com p.24
m) Juice Team/Shutterstock.com p.25
n) Lex-art/Shutterstock.com p.29
o) Blend Images/Shutterstock.com p.31
p) Ifong/Shutterstock.com p.32
q) Daxiao Productions/Shutterstock.com p.34
r) Malyugin/Shutterstock.com p.36
s) Pikselstock/Shutterstock.com p.37
t) Peter Bernik/Shutterstock.com p.39
u) Tmcphotos/Shutterstock.com p.40
v) Luis Louro/ Shutterstock.com p.42
w) Elena Elisseeva/Shutterstock.com p.44

x) Wavebreakmedia/Shutterstock.com p.45
y) IVY PHOTOS/Shutterstock.com p.46
z) Johan Larson/Shutterstock.com p.48
aa) Wavebreakmedia/Shutterstock.com p.49
bb) George Dolgikh/Shutterstock.com p.51
cc) Lucas Gojda/Shutterstock.com p.52
dd) Phil Date/Shutterstock.com p.54
ee) LuckyImages/Shutterstock.com p.55
ff) Photosani/Shutterstock.com p.58
gg) Filipe Frazao/Shutterstock.com p.59
hh) Pryzmat/Shutterstock.com p.62
ii) Luengchopan/Shutterstock.com p.64
jj) Michaeljung/Shutterstock.com p.83

Made in the USA
Middletown, DE
24 April 2017